Advance Praise from Experts

Anthony V. D'Amico, MD, PhD
Harvard Medical School, Professor of Radiation Oncology
Dana-Farber Cancer Institute, Chief, Division of Genitourinary Oncology

"*The Prostate Cancer Owner's Manual* is an outstanding and comprehensive resource that will be valuable for men and their families for years to come.

Dr. Haynes and Mr. Miles provide so much understandable information for so many about this debilitating and potentially deadly disease.

As authors, they did a terrific job in writing this book and should be thanked for sharing their commitments to inform others."

Dr. D'Amico is a professor of radiation oncology at Harvard Medical School and the chief of Genitourinary Radiation Oncology at the Brigham and Women's Hospital and Dana-Farber Cancer Institute.

He received his PhD in radiation physics from the Massachusetts Institute of Technology in 1986 and his MD from the University of Pennsylvania in 1990, where he also served as a resident and then chief resident in 1994.

He has gained international recognition for his work in detection, staging, and treatment of prostate cancer, with over 140 peer-reviewed articles published. He also has coedited four textbooks in urologic oncology. His prostate cancer research is funded by federal grants from the National Institutes of Health, National Cancer Institute, Department of Defense, and Massachusetts Department of Public Health.

Mark Pomerantz, MD
Harvard Medical School, Assistant Professor of Medicine
Dana-Farber Cancer Institute's Lank Center for Genitourinary Oncology

"I am very positive about the *Prostate Cancer Owner's Manual* because patients need to know what may lie ahead for them, and this book spells that out.

Mr. Miles and Dr. Haynes don't mince words. They see the problems and decisions patients face. They tell it as it is. They say what they believe based on their research and personal experiences.

The book says what patients need to hear; it is relevant, important, and straight-forward. This will be a good read for all patients, and people close to them."

Dr. Mark Pomerantz is a medical oncologist at the Dana-Farber Cancer Institute. He received his undergraduate degree from Yale University and his medical degree from Stanford University.

He trained in Internal Medicine at Boston's Brigham and Women's Hospital, then pursued a fellowship in medical oncology at the Dana-Farber Cancer Institute.

Dr. Pomerantz received his postdoctoral training in cancer genetics with Dr. Matthew Freedman at the Dana-Farber Cancer Institute and the Broad Institute of Harvard and Massachusetts Institute of Technology.

He is on the faculty of the Dana-Farber Cancer Institute's Lank Center for Genitourinary Oncology.

Sharon Bober, PhD, Senior Psychologist
Harvard Medical School, Assistant Professor of Psychology
Dana-Farber Cancer Institute's Psychosocial Oncology Program
Director, Dana-Farber's Sexual Health Program

> "Dr. Haynes and Mr. Miles perform a great service for readers of *The Prostate Cancer Owner's Manual* when they draw attention to the fact that palliative care is not just about death and dying. It is also about comprehensive symptom management in treating prostate cancer.
>
> I also appreciate their acknowledging the importance of the mind/body/spirit connection and their focus on intimacy and communication.
>
> For the majority of men, the prostate cancer experience is often transformative. Patients and partners can discover that 'having sex' is a flexible experience, not just a narrow focus on penile/penetrative intercourse. It is great to be happy with intimacy!"

Dr. Sharon Bober is the founder and director of the Sexual Health Program at Dana-Farber Cancer Institute in Boston, a senior psychologist, and an assistant professor of psychiatry at Harvard Medical School. Her specialties include adult psychosocial oncology, cancer survivorship, and sexual health.

Dr. Bober works with Dana-Farber's Psychosocial Oncology Program, which is part of the Department of Psychosocial Oncology and Palliative Care. She specializes in helping cancer patients and their families maintain the best quality of life during and after treatment. In this capacity, she helps them cope with emotional stress, including anxiety, depression, and changes in their thinking and behavior.

The Prostate Cancer
Owner's Manual

The Prostate Cancer Owner's Manual

What You Need to Know About Diagnosis, Treatment, and Survival

Harley A. Haynes, MD
and Richard M. Miles

in consultation with
Anthony V. D'Amico, MD, PhD, Oncologist
Mark Pomerantz, MD, Oncologist
Sharon Bober, PhD, Psychologist

ROWMAN & LITTLEFIELD
Lanham • Boulder • New York • London

Published by Rowman & Littlefield
An imprint of The Rowman & Littlefield Publishing Group, Inc.
4501 Forbes Boulevard, Suite 200, Lanham, Maryland 20706
www.rowman.com

6 Tinworth Street, London SE11 5AL, United Kingdom

British Library Cataloguing in Publication Information Available

Library of Congress Cataloging-in-Publication Data
Names: Haynes, Harley A., 1938- author; Miles, Richard M., 1946- author.
Title: The prostate cancer owner's manual : what you need to know about
    diagnosis, treatment, and survival / Richard M. Miles & Harley A.
    Haynes, M.D. ; in consultation with Anthony V. D'Amico, M.D., Ph.D.,
    Oncologist, Mark Pomerantz, M.D., Oncologist, Sharon Bober, Ph.D.,
    Psychologist.
Description: Lanham : Rowman & Littlefield Publishers, [2021] | Includes
    bibliographical references and index.
Identifiers: LCCN 2020056331 (print) | LCCN 2020056332 (ebook) | ISBN
    9781538153321 (cloth) | ISBN 9781538153338 (epub)
Subjects: LCSH: Prostate—Cancer.
Classification: LCC RC280.P7 M 2021 (print) | LCC RC280.P7 (ebook) | DDC
    616.99/463—dc23
LC record available at https://lccn.loc.gov/2020056331
LC ebook record available at https://lccn.loc.gov/2020056332

WHY WE WROTE THIS BOOK

We dedicate *The Prostate Cancer Owner's Manual* to all the men with prostate cancer—and those who might develop it. The fact that we've "been there, done that" has provided us with real-world knowledge of prostate cancer that we wish share with others.

This is similar to looking at an object from the inside out, versus looking from the outside in. It is the same object but viewed from a quite different perspective: From the perspective of a patient versus that of a doctor.

Therefore, *we* provide personal insights, independent facts, different perspectives of ongoing controversies about prostate cancer, extensive facts about the disease, its treatment, and a man's possible physiological and emotional reactions to the disease. Therefore, *The Prostate Cancer Owner's Manual* is very much a book written *for prostate cancer patients*, and it is dedicated to them.

We firmly believe that men deserve to know what's ahead for them in their battle with prostate cancer. We also believe that men and their families must learn and understand this information so that they can be prepared for what they may confront—and not be surprised by the changes in their bodies and minds. As the cliché goes, "forewarned is forearmed."

Contents

Introduction

THE AMAZING VASTNESS OF OUR AUDIENCE

We believe that prostate cancer is treated too lightly by many people, dismissed as a relatively rare—though inconvenient—disease. The following statistics, however, prove that such a cavalier attitude is grossly incorrect.

- Prostate cancer is the second most common form of cancer among American men, surpassed only by skin cancer, with 191,930 new cases diagnosed each year, for a total of 3.1 million cases.[1]
- Prostate cancer is one of the most prevalent malignant diseases among men. A new case is diagnosed about every three-and-a-half minutes and affects one in six men in their lifetime, according to the National Institutes of Health (NIH).
- Over 2.9 million American men, called "survivors," now live with prostate cancer or its post-treatment conditions.
- Every sixteen minutes in the United States, or more than ninety-one times a day, a man dies from prostate cancer. The total number of deaths in 2020 was 33,300.

Despite these truly powerful statistics, few men know much about this disease, the screening that is available to detect it, the risks of screening and not screening, how the disease is treated, and the radical changes in their bodily functions and their sexual abilities that result from many prostate cancer treatments.

Even worse, few men know that they will surely die from prostate cancer if it is allowed to spread, or metastasize, to other parts of the body. Even if a man beats death by prostate cancer, a metastasized cancer will require lifelong treatment with life-altering consequences.

As one urologist at Boston's Dana-Farber Cancer Institute (DFCI) quipped, "We don't want patients to get freaked out by the possible side-effects of the various treatments and simply not be tested. That could lead to a potentially terrible outcome for which there is no cure."

Indeed, that outcome could be fatal. Another DFCI doctor suggests that even when some men are told "the whole truth" about the disease, they ignore it or deny it. One truth about prostate cancer treatment is that men who undergo surgery, chemical treatment, or radiation therapy are almost assured of developing some form of incontinence and/or impotence.

Dr. Sharon Bober, a Dana-Farber psychologist who specializes in working with men dealing with the impact of prostate cancer, related a story about one of her patient's reaction.[2] During an early meeting with a patient, she warned him that, "Some men find that any incontinence—especially fecal incontinence—is more problematic than impotence."

"Oh, really!" the skeptical patient replied.

A year later, however, when fecal incontinence—as well as impotence—had become part of the same man's daily life, he admitted his naïveté and told Dr. Bober that he finally understood how urinary and/or fecal incontinence can easily trump impotence. That fact, that incontinence can "trump" impotence, shows the significant impact that prostate cancer treatment can have on a man's life, his psyche, and his behavior. Since incontinence, both urinary and fecal, is so common among prostate cancer patients, it will be mentioned several times in this book. Therefore, we believe that it is wise for readers to get a solid understanding of the condition and how it can progress.

Simply stated, incontinence—either urinary, fecal, or both—is the inability to control all or part of your elimination of urine or fecal matter. The condition may be light and sporadic, or regular and almost continuous. You can imagine for yourself how problematic such a condition can be. Because many men often don't get adequate information about prostate cancer, however, they benignly live their lives seduced by the reassuring phrase, "more men die with the disease than from it."[3]

To make matters worse, some men are swayed into inaction because they are told that unnecessary, time-consuming, and possibly costly screening may result in unnecessary "over-testing" and thus "over-treating."

This conundrum of whether or not to test—and when and how often—will also be dealt with in greater detail later in this book.

One bright spot about prostate cancer, however, is the fact that when it's detected and treated at an early stage, a man's chances of living to a natural death are virtually 100 percent. While his life may be fraught with physical and psychological problems, these are usually better than the alternative. These and other quality of life issues are discussed as well.

If the prostate cancer is not detected early and is allowed to spread (or metastasize), then a man's quality of life—until he dies of it—is often characterized by sexual impotence, urinary and/or fecal incontinence, loss of energy, muscle strength and stamina, and a plethora of other physiological challenges.

Our goal, therefore, is to provide men with an authoritative, easy-to-read "manual" that helps them understand prostate cancer, how it can change their bodies and minds, and the overall quality of life implications they will be required to face.

Section 1

FIRST THINGS FIRST

1

This Is How It All Begins

Your first experience with prostate cancer can be purely accidental, resulting from a routine physical exam by your physician; or it can be dramatic. In either case, when you walk out of your doctor's office with the news that you might have prostate cancer you are shocked, frightened, and bewildered.

You didn't know you had such a problem; you don't know how you got it; and regardless of what your doctor said, you're not sure what your prostate cancer means for the rest of your life, for your family, for your job. Everything! But, hopefully, this chapter will assure you based on our experiences, our outcomes, and the fact that we are both still alive. Life does exist after prostate cancer, at least for most men.

I'm Richard Miles, and my journey into the medical and emotional maze of prostate cancer began as simply as yours may have—with my annual physical. Dr. Harley Haynes' experience began in a much more dramatic fashion, with blood in his urine.

In my case, my personal physician was highly regarded by his colleagues and other patients at Boston's Brigham and Women's Hospital. He loved his profession, his patients, and his family. He often talked about watching *SpongeBob SquarePants* on TV with his two young children. But that's the type of person my personal physician was. When he was alive, he cared very deeply about his patients and his family.

Several years ago, I expected my annual physical to end as they always had before, with something like: "All's well; but you might want to get a little more exercise and keep new pounds off." But that routine send-off was not to be for me. "Richard," my physician said,

"I'm afraid I have to tell you that your blood tests show you have an elevated PSA. That's a Prostate Specific Antigen, and when it is as high as yours—which appears to be about 8.25—there's a chance that you have prostate cancer. That's good and bad. It is good because you are relatively young. And it is bad because you are relatively young."

I can't say that I was devastated, but I was bewildered. I didn't know what an "elevated PSA" really meant. Cancer's bad, but I had had skin cancers before, and Harley Haynes, then my dermatologist, had taken care of it. There wasn't much to those cancers, so how much worse could prostate cancer be?

But my doctor's manner had changed. Prostate cancer. What is that really?

How do I get rid of it? Surgery? Really? How bad could that be?

Obviously, it wasn't good, or my doctor wouldn't have looked or sounded so glum. He was never glum; he was always a happy guy.

But what did today's experience really mean?

Then, he began his paced and understandable explanation.

"First," he said, "I want you to see an oncologist to get his assessment. I'll set that up. At the same time, we are going to choose one of a couple of very good prostate cancer surgeons that I'm familiar with and set a time to remove your prostate. That's assuming, of course, that your urologist believes that's the way to go. But we want to get you into the urologist—and on a surgeon's schedule—so we can move quickly if your PSA indicates what I believe it does."

What's all this? I thought. Oncologist? Surgery? Speed? Need to act fast? What is going on here? I was expecting a routine physical and "Have a nice day."

I didn't know anything about an elevated PSA, much less real honest-to-God surgery, then chemical therapy and a series of radiation treatments. What radiation!? No one had said anything about radiation! What does this all mean?

It all meant a lot, and that day and the days that followed would change my life and my world forever, and not by just a little bit!

That was eighteen years ago; I was 56 at the time. As for Dr. Harley Haynes—my former dermatologist and now coauthor and fellow PC survivor—his diagnosis was only five years ago, and the impact of that discovery has grown over time. It didn't hit him like a bolt of lightning as it hit me.

You may read articles and other books that say, "Oh, well. You'll get over the treatments. And you'll adapt to your new life; it's not so bad." Well, we're here to tell you that your life *will* change!

Harley's prostate cancer discovery was quite different than mine, and it took a few weeks to come to full recognition of it by both Harley and his physician. What follows are his own words about his own experience of being diagnosed with prostate cancer.

One day I noticed a bit of blood in my urine. I was seventy-seven at the time, and the event wasn't particularly upsetting to me; after all, it was just that one episode and not particularly unexpected for a man of my age, so I continued my medical practice and, basically, forgot about the incident. Everything was fine for several weeks.

Then I noticed that I had blood in my urine almost every time I went to the bathroom. I called my primary care doctor, and he reassured me that a lot of men my age have that. But, he added, to make sure that everything was okay, he'd have a look.

So, I rearranged my patient schedule, and a couple of days later I was the patient—a role reversal, you might say. My doctor did a digital rectal exam (DRE) as a first step. "I don't feel anything unusual," he said, "but let's get an expert's opinion. I'll make an appointment for you with Dr. Harrison (not his real name), who is a urologist, and we'll see what he finds, if anything." Dr. Harrison also performed a DRE, and he indeed felt a nodule. He immediately scheduled me for a full-scale needle biopsy of my prostate later that week.

That Friday he took six biopsies, three on each side of my prostate. Since the samples had to be examined by a lab, I would not know the results until Monday. I'm the inquisitive sort, however, so when I got to work at the hospital that Monday morning, I logged into my computer account, looked up my own pathology report, and discovered—Oh my God!—I did indeed had cancer, with a Gleason score of 9, and the cancer had invaded both lobes of my prostate. No wonder I was having blood in my urine!

As I was trying to internalize what all of this meant, I was sitting at my desk, behind the computer screen, planning to have a conversation with the young trainee who was waiting patiently outside my office. Since my door was open, I motioned him in, but he could tell by the look on my face that something was wrong. He thought it was something bad *about him* that he was about to learn, but in fact, it was something very bad *about me*. I dismissed him without ever explaining why he was there or what I had just discovered about me.

I was thinking, "How could this be?" Initially, my concerns were about treating some form of low-grade cancer, and now, my God, I'm wondering if I am going to live. I was really shaken up! I certainly didn't expect that pathology report.

I thought back to my personal physician's assessment. Well, that was clearly wrong. The only good thing was that the event reaffirmed my belief in specialists, of which I was one, a dermatologist. The urologist knew what he was looking for and also knew when he found it. So he set me up for a series of other tests. One of them was a rectal MRI (Magnetic Resonance Imaging) performed by a young resident, who explained to me that it was a routine exam. But it was anything but; it felt as if he was jamming a Volkswagen up my rear. I grabbed onto the sides of the examining table so tightly that my arm muscles were sore for days.

Nothing good came from that experience. The tests showed that my cancer had escaped from the prostate capsule and invaded the sphincter. That was the reason for the blood in my urine. With that result, my primary care physician expressed dismay at those results, but referred me to a genitourinary oncologist, one of the top internal experts at Dana-Farber Cancer Institute, where I also practiced—as well as at the Brigham and Women's Hospital.

For my first meeting with him, my wife accompanied me, as the doctor had requested. (I would recommend that to everyone in this situation. It is very important to have a spouse fully informed so that she knows what to expect in the months and years to come.)

The night after our meeting with the oncologist, we went to bed, and I broke down sobbing. I held my wife tightly until I fell asleep. I fell apart and cried only one other time during my five-year prostate cancer ordeal, and that was a couple of years ago.

My wife and I went to our church, across the street from our home, and followed the stations of the cross. When we got to the place where I was supposed to hammer a nail into the cross, I broke down sobbing; I was so grateful that I had a chance to be cured as opposed to dying like Jesus. At least I wasn't going die from the cancer.

It was incredibly meaningful and a life-changing event. Nothing seemed quite the same as it had before. Compared to dying, impotence and incontinence aren't that bad. Not that I am comfortable with them, but they're better than death.

WHO IS AT RISK FOR PROSTATE CANCER?

According to the Centers for Disease Control and Prevention, "All men are at risk for prostate cancer. Out of every 100 American men, about 13 will get prostate cancer during their lifetime, and about 2 to 3 men will die from prostate cancer. The most common risk factor is age. The older a man is, the greater the chance of getting prostate cancer."[1]

But some men are at more increased risk than others for getting prostate cancer.

You are at increased risk of getting, or dying, from prostate cancer if you are an African American or have a family history of prostate cancer. And men—regardless of race or nationality—who have a father, son, or brother who had prostate cancer are also at increased risk for developing the disease.

Men who are neither African American nor have a family history of prostate cancer are at average risk.

2

Your First Questions Are Answered, But . . .

Your initial experience with the medical profession with respect to prostate cancer is likely to be frustrating—if it hasn't already been. You probably will have many more questions than answers.

The short answer to the most-asked question is, "You are more likely to die with prostate cancer" than from it. That, however, greatly oversimplifies the disease.

The vagaries of modern medicine, and your own urge to know, will push you to the edge. Therefore, you will go exploring on your own, and that can be dangerous because it likely will include searching the internet and watching YouTube *videos.*

These can both be fun sources of information, but a close examination of YouTube *reveals that there is often an inverse relationship between a video's popularity and the accuracy of its prostate cancer information.*

We would ask, therefore, "Do you want YouTube *to be your doctor?"*
When you want giggles, watch YouTube; *when you want serious medical information, however, you need to get it from your doctor and other respected cancer authorities.*

We were no different than you and the many other men who have received the unwelcome and alarming news: "Your PSA test indicates that you may have prostate cancer." Even worse is when your doctor tells you such an indication from your PSA test (prostate-specific antigen) results can only be confirmed by a "work-up," which means the procedures done to arrive at a diagnosis, including family and medical history, laboratory tests, X-rays, perhaps a digital rectal exam (DRE), and most likely more lab tests. The frustration and anxiety begin!

It is an unfilled blank space not knowing if you have prostate cancer, not knowing what's going to happen to you, and when. And, of course, an army of abstract numbers and terms will pummel you, almost all of which are couched in conditional terms like "may," "might," "could," "if when," and the inevitable, "we don't know."

We have been there, too, and we're pretty certain that among your first questions will be:

- Am I going to die?
- How long do I have to live?
- What will be my quality of life?

As is often the case with doctors and other healthcare professionals, they may not answer directly any of those three very basic and very important questions. But we will. In the following chapters, and we will answer those questions and many more:

- Am I going to die? Yes, eventually. We all do.
- How long do I have to live? If you discover your prostate cancer early in its development, you probably will have a long life. If you discover it after it has spread—metastasized—the prognosis is more problematic and dependent on how old you are at the time of diagnosis.
- What will be my quality of life? If you do have prostate cancer and it is detected before it metastasizes, your life will change, but in most cases, patients can manage around the changes that will come. If the cancer has begun to metastasize, it is a grimmer story, which we will discuss in detail further.

While those are genuine answers—even though every prostate cancer case is unique—we understand the uncertainties you are facing, and we will seek to provide you with the answers you need to understand the implications of your prostate cancer and its impact on your future.

Now, let's deal with information from the internet and *YouTube*.

YouTube is clearly a more entertaining source of information; after all, it presents videos, and you don't have to read weighty—and sometimes obtuse—sentences that themselves need explaining! Nonetheless, information about prostate cancer and its detection, treatment, and outcomes are readily available on the internet from many reputable hospitals, institutions, and associations (we have listed some excellent websites at the end of this book), but it is a different situation. While these commercial sites are largely designed to provide you with entertainment, their information about prostate cancer can sometimes be useful in providing different points of view that you might not readily get elsewhere. You must be very cautious, however, especially about the following considerations:

* Timeliness of the information you're reading and viewing: Is it current?
* Accuracy and balance of the information: Who is providing it?
* Commercial motives of the information provider: Does the provider have more of a financial stake than a medical or ethical stake in your medical decisions?

If you think that *YouTube* as a source of serious information is a medium of little consequence with only modest influence, let's look at some amazing statistics.

* *YouTube* CEO Susan Wojcicki was quoted in the online publication *The Verge* saying that it has "1.8 billion registered users watching videos on the platform each month, not counting anyone who's watching without an account."[1]
* "Almost 5 billion videos are watched on *YouTube* every single day," according to the February 26, 2020, edition of *MerchDope.*
* MedPageToday reported on November 28, 2018, that an analysis of 51 prostate cancer videos showed that 73 percent . . . provided fair to poor information, and 69 percent exhibited a clear bias in favor of screening or treatment. Since 2008, there has been a "more than 1,000-fold increase in *YouTube* videos" about prostate cancer, but "there are limited data on the nature and quality of current information."[2]

Dr. Stacy Loeb and her colleagues at New York University's Langone Medical Center conducted "the largest, most comprehensive examination of prostate cancer information on *YouTube* to date," and the alarming and disconcerting results were published in the November 27, 2018, edition of *European Urology.*[3]

Dr. Loeb cautioned readers that the "*YouTube* videos about prostate cancer contained biased or poor-quality information" and that *the popularity of a video has no relationship to the quality of its content.* Thus, "a greater number of views and thumbs up on *YouTube* do not mean that the information is trustworthy." A summary of her research findings shows the following alarming statistics that you should consider if you choose to view the *YouTube* content on prostate cancer.

- The *YouTube* videos in the researchers' sample had up to an amazing 1.3 million views each, with an average individual viewership of over forty-five thousand, yet Dr. Loeb writes, "The overall quality of information was moderate."
- The *YouTube* videos leaned heavily toward positive outcomes, with 73 percent describing benefits but just over 53 percent describing the harm of various actions and treatments.
- Of particular interest was that "only 50% [of the videos viewed] promoted shared decision-making as recommended in current guidelines"—and were strongly supported by us. (Read about joint decision-making and related topics in the section "Managing my Prostate Cancer Decisions" later in this book.)
- One of Dr. Loeb's most damning findings was that a total of 115 videos—or 77 percent of the 150 examined—"contained potentially mis-informative and/or biased content within the video or comments section."
- Unfortunately, and ironically, the worse a video's factual medical quality, the higher was its viewer engagement. Thus, "a significant negative correlation [exists] between scientific quality and viewer engagement."
- While medicine is a complex area of endeavor with unique language often difficult to understand, "only 54% of the [*YouTube*] videos defined medical terms, and few provided summaries or references" to help viewers better understand the video presentation.

Dr. Loeb also noted that, "The comments section underneath some videos contained advertising and peer-to-peer medical advice." As the saying goes: consider the source.

To their credit, however, "most videos had clear objectives, a logical flow of information, and good audio quality." Even with those

Who Is at Risk for Prostate Cancer?

- All men are at risk for prostate cancer. Out of every 100 American men, about thirteen will get prostate cancer during their lifetime, and about two to three men will die from prostate cancer.
- The most common risk factor is age. The older a man is, the greater his chance of getting prostate cancer.
- Some men are at increased risk for prostate cancer. You are at increased risk for getting or dying from prostate cancer if you are African American or have a family history of prostate cancer. Men who have a father, son, or brother who had prostate cancer also are at increased risk for getting prostate cancer.
- Men who are not African American and do not have a family history of prostate cancer are at average risk.

Source: Centers for Disease Control and Prevention, "Who Is at Risk for Prostate Cancer?" August 8, 2020, https://www.cdc.gov/cancer/prostate/basic_info/risk_factors.htm.

plusses, "few [of the *YouTube* videos about prostate cancer] discussed multiple options, provided sources, or summarized the information. Only approximately half of the videos defined medical terms, divided information into sections, or addressed users directly when describing actions."

Perhaps most unnerving was the fact that viewers were using the video service as an online doctor: "We also noted significant persuasion of users to pursue guideline-discordant treatment or unproven natural remedies by videos and/or social interactions with other users."

Dr. Loeb's group report concludes with this cautionary note:

In summary, many popular videos about PC [prostate cancer] on *YouTube* lack key elements of shared decision-making and contain biased content. The significant inverse relationship between expert ratings of information quality and the popularity of videos on *YouTube* is highly concerning because of the facilitation of wide dissemination of potentially mis-informative content.

Chapter 2

IN OUR OPINION. . .

We believe that YouTube *is an entertaining and sometimes accurate informative source, but it should not be relied on for authoritative information about prostate cancer about which life, death, and quality of life decisions are made.*

Prostate cancer is a very serious and often elusive disease that will materially change your life, and we believe that it is more than a little bit risky to put your life, and the quality of your life, in the hands of an unknown video producer whose knowledge and motives are not known to you.

YouTube *may provide a foundation for raising important questions, and those questions should be presented to your healthcare team, which includes your oncologist, your palliative care specialist, your spouse, and others.*

The final question is: "Do you want YouTube *to be your doctor?"*

3

Let's Get Prostate Cancer in Perspective

Prostate cancer is not only the second most common cancer in men, after skin cancer, but also the second leading cause of cancer death among men. African American men and men with a family history of prostate cancer have a higher chance of developing the disease. In 2020 alone, 191,930 American men were diagnosed with prostate cancer and about 33,300 died from it.[1] While the prostate cancer number is large, you should remember that there were about 157,000,000 men in the United States at the end of 2016. The total US population was about 320,000,000.

In the following chapters, we deal with what you should look for, the tests that you may need to determine the extent of your prostate cancer, and the treatments that will likely be suggested for its remediation. We address the question, "What did I do to deserve this?"—age, genetics, lifestyle, etc., in the final chapters of this book. What you did to deserve this is largely an academic question; what you do now that you have it is the most important question.

As an American man, you have one chance in nine of being diagnosed with prostate cancer, but the risk of dying from prostate cancer is pretty slim. Indeed, many prostate cancers often advance so slowly that they are not detected during a man's lifetime, only during an autopsy. "The men most affected by prostate cancer are older than 50," writes the website Aging.com.[2] The following is a list of a man's chances of developing prostate cancer at different age ranges.

- Before 50, 1 in 403
- Between 50 and 59, 1 in 58

- Between 60 and 69, 1 in 21
- Between 70 and 79, 1 in 14

Thus, those numbers are the foundation for the often-used rationalization that "You are more likely to die with prostate cancer than of it." It is a phrase, however, that is "a wolf in sheep's clothing," as you will discover as you read further.

These seemingly positive facts should not minimize your concern about the actual risk of developing prostate cancer, the need for early detection, and your considerable risks associated with overtreatment or, worse, late detection. Late detection means that the cancer has spread to adjacent tissue, thus spreading to other parts of your body; that is, it has metastasized.

While medical experts disagree on the actual need for or the frequency of prostate cancer testing screening, "there is consensus that the longer a cancer is allowed to exist, the more aggressive it becomes and the more threatening it is to your quality of life. Therefore, one critical question according to Dr. Mark Pomerantz at the Dana-Farber Cancer Institute in Boston is: "Are you old enough to outlive the cancer?"

According to the medical journal *UpToDate*, "The five-year relative survival among men with cancer confined to the prostate (localized or with just a regional spread) is 100 percent, compared with 29.3 percent among those diagnosed with distant metastases. While men with advanced-stage disease may benefit from some advanced treatments, their tumors are generally not curable."[3] Webster defines metastases as "the spread of a disease-producing agent . . . from the initial or primary site of disease to another part of the body."

IN OUR OPINION. . .

We believe that prostate cancer should be given the attention and respect it rightfully deserves. We also believe that the facts speak for themselves: "For all sites combined, the cancer incidence rate is 20% higher in men than in women, while the cancer death rate is 40% higher," according to 2017 statistics published in the journal CA: A Cancer Journal for Clinicians. We believe that this is the result of a combination of at least two factors: 1. A generalized form of silent "sexism," and 2. Patients' ignorance of the environmental subtleties of men and women in social environments.

As to the first factor, the volatile topic of "sexism," here's an example. When friends and family are informed that cousin Elizabeth has breast cancer, the common reaction is along the lines of: "Oh, my God. The poor baby. How's she going to cope with that?" When friends and family are informed that their cousin Fred has prostate cancer, however, the common reaction is along the lines of: "Oh, jeez, but Fred will be okay. He's a strong guy. Besides, no one dies of prostate cancer these days; they die with it."

What is the difference in these two reactions?

First, let's look at the situation from the sexist's perspective. It is unlikely that Elizabeth's breast cancer will render her sexually impotent. In the vast majority of cases, the Elizabeths of the world will be able to continue having normal sexual intercourse.

By contrast, Fred's prostate cancer could easily render him sexually impotent, making normal sexual intercourse impossible. We believe that the likely outcomes are dramatic and should be noted.

Second is the ignorance that goes beyond the mere physiological differences. Historically, women talk with other women about their personal, physical, and psychological conditions: what's happening, how they feel, perhaps even the quality of their relationships. Men, by contrast, generally don't talk about their feelings or emotional reactions; that would be weak and unmanly. Men also don't talk about their sexuality or complain about their lack of sexual prowess.

As we noted earlier, 33,300 American men died of prostate cancer in 2020. We believe that one reason prostate cancer does not get the respect it deserves is because so many people, including doctors, propagate the notion that, "Men don't die of prostate cancer, they die with it." The death toll shows how wrong that is.

4

What Are the Symptoms of Prostate Trouble?

First, you should understand that there are several different types of prostate cancer, but the most common—which make up about 95 to 99 percent of cases—are considered adenocarcinomas.[1] (You can read about the different types of prostate cancer, and how each behaves, at ProstateCancer .net in the section called Types of Prostate Cancer.*)*

Despite the varieties, "the challenge in treating prostate cancer is that it can either behave like a pussycat—growing slowly and unlikely to cause problems in a man's lifetime—or a tiger—spreading aggressively and requiring urgent treatment," according to Prof. Malcolm Mason of Cancer Research UK.

The problem, he explains, is that "at the moment we have no reliable way to distinguish them."[2] Nonetheless, men should be on guard for the symptoms for prostate cancer because all types are potential killers.

Symptoms to look for include blood in urine or semen, a weak or interrupted urinary stream, inability to urinate standing up, and experiencing a painful sensation while urinating or ejaculating—among others detailed on the following pages.

While prostate cancer is one of the most common types of male cancers, in its early stages, it usually exhibits no symptoms. Indeed, the American Cancer Society (ACS) states that many early problems "are more likely to be caused by something other than prostate cancer."[3] For instance, "Trouble urinating is much more often caused by benign prostatic hyperplasia (BPH), a noncancerous growth of the prostate." Other potential signs that prostate cancer may be developing include the following:[4]

- Urination problems that include a slow or weak stream or the need to urinate more often, especially at night
- Blood in the urine or semen
- Difficulty achieving an erection
- Loss of bladder control
- Pain in the hips, back, chest, or other boney areas that may indicate the cancer has spread, or metastasized, to the bones
- Weakness or numbness in thighs, legs, or feet

While some of these symptoms may appear in prostate diseases that are not prostate cancer, it's important to tell your healthcare provider about them so that you and he or she can determine their causes and settle on an appropriate treatment, if one is needed. The three most common prostate diseases in order of frequency are:[5]

1. Prostatitis
2. Benign Prostatic Hyperplasia
3. Prostate cancer

PROSTATITIS

Prostatitis is a prostate inflammation that can be caused by a bacterial infection. "Men of all ages can get prostatitis, and it can occur in any size prostate (enlarged or not)," according to *Web*MD. Symptoms of prostatitis include:

- Urination difficulty
- Pain or a burning sensation during urination
- Frequent urination, especially at night
- Chills and fever accompanying urinating problems

BENIGN PROSTATIC HYPERPLASIA

BPH is a very common noncancerous enlargement of the prostate gland, which rarely causes noticeable symptoms in men younger than forty years old.

According to the American Urological Association (AUA), about half of men between ages fifty-one and sixty, and up to 90 percent of men older than eighty have BPH. Its symptoms include:

* Urination difficulty, difficulty getting a stream started
* An urge to urinate even when your bladder is empty
* Frequent urination, especially at night
* A weak or intermittent stream as well as a sense of incomplete emptying when urinating

PROSTATE CANCER

Early-stage prostate cancer usually does not exhibit symptoms; however, as it progresses, symptoms may begin to appear. Dana-Farber's Dr. Mark Pomerantz's research focuses on the factors associated with cancer risk, with an emphasis on prostate cancer. While prostate cancer develops in the setting of many environmental and inherited risk factors, Dr. Pomerantz has focused since 2006 on examining the inherited component of the disease.

"Clearly we know that one early indication of the possible existence of prostate cancer comes from looking at one's inheritance: Did another member of the patient's family have prostate cancer. If the answer is 'Yes' we know that the patient has an elevated chance of developing the disease," said Dr. Pomerantz. "Unfortunately," he added, "the mechanisms in which the inherited factors predispose a man to disease are unknown."

Working closely with clinicians, biostatisticians, and epidemiologists at Dana-Farber and MIT's Broad Institute, he is actively deciphering this mechanism in an attempt to define the underpinnings of prostate cancer risk. We discuss in more detail the inheritance risk later in this book.

As to the stealthy nature of prostate cancer, the ACS warns that, "There are no warning signs of early prostate cancer. Once a tumor causes the prostate gland to swell, or once cancer spreads beyond the prostate, the following symptoms may happen."[6]

- Urination problems that include a slow or weak stream or the need to urinate more often, especially at night
- Inability to urinate
- Weak or interrupted flow of urine (dribbling)
- Painful or burning urination
- Painful ejaculation
- Difficulty achieving an erection
- Blood in the urine or semen
- Weakness or numbness in thighs, legs, or feet

The ACS points out that "These are not symptoms of the cancer itself; instead, they are caused by the blockage from the cancer growth in the prostate." While that is the case, it is important to note that symptoms can also be caused by a noncancerous enlarged prostate or by a urinary tract infection.

IN OUR OPINION. . .

We agree with the American Cancer Society that many symptoms of prostate cancer can be exhibited by other male problems. Nonetheless, we suggest that a call to your doctor for an appointment to determine the actual cause of your condition is prudent. Prostate problems are very serious business and are not to be toyed with.

As we will point out in subsequent pages and sections, early and accurate detection of prostate cancer is critical to your health and, indeed, your life. To brush off the symptoms with the hackneyed phrase that "men die with prostate cancer, not of it" is dangerous. It can be a deadly situation, and it is much wiser to be safe than sorry.

Having offered such advice, we also urge you to

1. *Be Cautious—You should be cautious because an inaccurate identification of prostate cancer can result in unnecessary treatment that likely will alter the rest of your life.*
2. *Seek Multiple Opinions—We believe in getting the opinions of more than one doctor, and you should have more than one test to identify the possible existence of the disease.*

3. *Seek Counseling—If you develop prostate cancer, we strongly believe that you and your partner or spouse should seek experienced, professional counseling. This will allow you both to better understand the disease, the implications of its treatment, and the way the rest of your life will likely change.*

5

The Importance of Early Screening and Diagnosis

Regular prostate-specific antigen (PSA) testing and screening can be costly, time consuming, and may not produce conclusive results—and it presents the opportunity to "overtreat." Yet, the opposite option—called watchful waiting or active surveillance—also offers considerable risks. You should also know that screening practices and their quality differ among medical professionals, institutions, and countries.

One medical opinion is that less testing, or active surveillance, is desirable because it reduces the risk of false positives, thus potentially eliminating unnecessary but very impactful treatments. Watchful waiting, however, runs the risk of the cancer metastasizing, which also has significant negative implications for quality of life.

Another opinion is that regular and cautious testing is needed to catch even the few prostate cancers that might otherwise escape and enable the least drastic treatment and possibly preventing metastasizing of the cancer.

On the following pages, you will find a considerable amount of information about various aspects of research and divergent (as well as controversial) professional opinions on prostate cancer testing. This is because testing is *the* initial building block for all that will follow in the process of identifying and treating your prostate cancer. Testing is critical to your treatment, your quality of life and, indeed, your very survival.

Prostate cancer screening may be *the* initial building block in determining the existence of a problem. However, "many studies show that men lack knowledge of prostate cancer screening, including the advantages and disadvantages of the PSA test. A few studies have assessed the frequency of discussion of the PSA test." One such study stated that "fewer than one-half of 304 tested men reported discussing the advantages and disadvantages of the test." In a Veterans Affairs setting, one researcher found that "two thirds of tested men recalled having the test, and 47 percent reported discussing its advantages and disadvantages," according to a September 4, 2006, article in the *Annals of Family Medicine.*

The subject of prostate testing seems quite controversial, with two side emerging: Test and Test Later. In the United States, two basic schools of thought exist regarding prostate cancer screening. One is espoused by the United States Preventive Service Task Force (USP-STF), a federally funded volunteer group that believes testing has been overdone and has produced many false positive results, causing overtreatment and negative psychological outcomes. It was created in 1984 as a well-respected group of sixteen experts representing internal medicine, family medicine, pediatrics, behavioral health, obstetrics/gynecology, and nursing.

With the advent of President Barack Obama's Affordable Care Act (ACA) in 2009, the "not particularly well known" USPSTF became recognized by the administration as a potentially influential voice in the practice of medicine. Therefore, to reduce its potential impact regarding medical diagnosis on public opinion, the USPSTF significantly reduced its review and publication of medical analysis and became an organization in which "politics would begin trumping science," according to Dr. Kenneth Lin, in a KevinMD.com article, "How Politics Have Weakened the USPSTF."[1] Dr. Lin is a specialist in internal medicine practicing in Arlington, Virginia, who says the USPSFT became "only a shadow of its independent self," and suggested that, "A Task Force that makes few waves is exactly what the (then current Obama) Administration want(ed)."[2]

The other side of the argument, expressed cautiously by the American Urological Association (AUA), suggests that testing helps catch prostate cancer before it metastasizes, rendering it incurable and virtually assuring death from prostate cancer if the man does not die from other causes first. Aware of the politics of prostate cancer testing, the AUA issued the following statement, in which it very cautiously endorses testing despite the USPSTF's position to the contrary.

The psychological impact of prostate cancer screening must be considered and viewed as a potential harm. . . . Along with the stress due to PSA screening and unnecessary biopsies, the diagnosis of prostate cancer alone may incite severe psychological stress with one study showing an increased rate of suicide and cardiovascular events in newly diagnosed men.

Potential harms must be carefully discussed with a man prior to embarking on a screening program and at each step of screening . . . [and that a] man should be given the information and the option of stopping based on his individual Quality of Life and longevity goals.[3]

The AUA adds that a "man should be given information" that includes counseling as he works his way through this medical challenge. (We discuss counseling opportunities—and the lack thereof—before, during, and after diagnosis and treatment in section 4 of this book. "The benefits of PSA screening merit careful consideration," according to a 2013 AUA paper, "Early Detection of Prostate Cancer." Screening is especially important in "decreasing the risk of metastatic disease."[4]

Since the advent of PSA screening, the incidence of advanced prostate cancer "has declined remarkably and death rates from prostate cancer, as reported in the National Cancer Database, have declined at the rate of 1% per year since 1990. Other data indicate similar declines in prostate cancer related mortality in the US."

The AUA pointedly notes:

In addition to seeing a decline in mortality, there is also an increase in disease incidence. This could reflect either greater screening practices or greater prevalence of true risk factors for prostate cancer in the population (e.g., changing dietary habits, increasing obesity rates, environmental toxins, etc.) or the advent of extended biopsy protocols that sample twice or more the number of cores than were being sampled in the early- to mid-1990s.

Given the paradox of rising incidence but falling mortality, it is highly unlikely that the rising prevalence is a factor that truly increases prostate cancer risk and could account for these findings.[5]

Indeed, the AUA believes that "The benefits of prostate cancer screening may extend beyond improving survival and could accrue from limiting disease morbidity arising from bladder outlet obstruction, hematuria, bone pain, etc." Obviously, reduction of disease morbidity results in an improved quality of life, not just an extension of life itself.

Two European studies also contribute to the belief in the efficacy of testing as a means of reducing advanced or metastasized prostate cancer. In data from the European Randomized Study of Screening for Prostate Cancer (ERSPC), the cumulative risk of metastatic disease at nine to eleven years of follow-up was 31 percent to 33 percent lower in the screened arm compared to the control arm. The Göteborg, Sweden, arm of that trial demonstrated a 56 percent reduction in the risk of metastatic disease. Most of this reduction was seen in cancers detected at the time of diagnosis in the screened arm. Göteborg is the Swedish name for the Anglicized name Gothenburg; however, Göteborg is the name the ERSPC uses, so we shall use it, too.

Mere monitoring in a watchful-waiting approach—as compared with treatment—leads to increased incidence of metastasis, wrote Dr. Anthony V. D'Amico, in *The New England Journal of Medicine* (*NEJM*). Dr. D'Amico is a radiation oncologist and the Chief of Genitourinary Radiation Oncology Program at the Dana-Farber/Brigham and Women's Cancer Center. He is also a professor in radiation oncology at Harvard Medical School.

TREATMENT OPTIONS

While "the best" initial approach to managing early low-risk and intermediate-risk prostate cancers remains unknown, existing clinical evidence suggests three treatment options, if he has a life expectancy of greater than ten years:

1. Active monitoring
2. Surgery
3. A combination of radiation, surgery, and hormone therapy

One fact is certain, however; mere PSA monitoring leads to increased metastasis of early prostate cancer, wrote Dr. D'Amico.

Therefore, to avoid metastatic prostate cancer and its negative quality-of-life effects, *monitoring should be considered only if the man has a life expectancy of less than ten years* (absent the impact of the prostate cancer), according to Dr. D'Amico.

If a man has a life expectancy greater than ten years, then he should feel free to select one of the listed three options. These options are available because there is no significant difference in the death rate between these types of treatment. To determine how we arrived at this conclusion, let's examine the outcomes associated with each of the three prostate cancer treatment regimes.

The results of active monitoring show that active men, those who selected the "active monitoring" route for dealing with prostate cancer, were more than twice as likely to have their cancer metastasize as compared to the men who were actually treated for the disease. The data shows the following:

- 6.3 cases per one thousand person-years for the "monitored" men versus 2.4 to 3.0 cases per one thousand person-years for the tested men.
- The numbers appear to be relatively small, but when extrapolated to the entire population, their significance increases. If you are among that group, the number is indeed significant.

In short, fewer men died from prostate cancer among those who received either surgery or a combination of radiation and ADT when compared to those men who selected "active monitoring." As noted earlier, the significance of this finding is that by choosing "active monitoring," more men will have metastases, which results in a significantly greater negative quality-of-life impact than from Androgen Deprivation Therapy (ADT). And if a man does not die of another cause, he will certainly die from metastatic prostate cancer.

To understand the significance of a decreased quality of life, please read the section "About Harold's Prostate Situation" later in this book. As with most things, there are multiple sides to any argument, and prostate cancer is no different. So it is with Dr. Deborah Kuban at the MD Anderson Cancer Center in Houston.

To confuse the issue even further, the British publication *Prostate Cancer UK* points out and passes the buck with the following statement: "Some people use names such as 'active monitoring' and 'wait and see' to describe both active surveillance and watchful waiting. These can mean different things to different people, so ask your doctor or nurse to explain exactly what they mean."

A March 2020 article in *MedNet News* reports that a 2004 to 2016 study by Dr. Kuban and others at the Houston hospital conducted among 4,451 men favored the course of "active surveillance" over surgery, radiation, or chemical treatment when a multidisciplinary environment existed.[6] A multidisciplinary approach, according to the article, found "typically in major cancer centers," involves a patient getting the opinions of multiple experts, rather than just seeing a series of urologists.

Dr. Kuban is quoted as stating that when the research began in 2004, about 10 percent of those men who tested positive for prostate cancer chose active surveillance. In 2016, the last year of our study, when the multidisciplinary approach was in full swing, 80 percent of the prostate cancer patients chose active surveillance.

The same *MedNet News* article cited a *Journal of Clinical Oncology* report from September 2012 that referenced a four-year study at the Massachusetts General Hospital. That study compared the outcomes of 701 men who participated in a multidisciplinary approach to treatment. At the outset of that study, 43 percent of the men who utilized such an approach chose active surveillance, compared to the 22 percent who chose active surveillance after consulting with a urologist or a radiation oncologist. "In the intervening years, the proportion of men opting for AS [active surveillance] had grown to 70%–80%." The implications of those numbers are clear and are restated later in this book: "Urologists and radiation oncologists [are biased] toward recommending their own tools." While this may be the case, the *MedNet News* article does not mention the age ranges of the men in the MD Anderson or the Mass General studies, which can have a significant influence on their outcomes.

The evidence shows that more men over the age of sixty-five were likely to die from prostate cancer if they chose "active monitoring" over treatment for prostate cancer. Because of the limited breadth of the study, however, this is considered "a near-significant" outcome, although it is nonetheless meaningful, especially if you are in that small percentage.

Dr. D'Amico says the determinate in choosing watchful waiting overactive intervention—or moving from watchful waiting into action—is the "velocity of the PSA," the rate of upward change of the PSA metric. A relatively stable PSA would suggest continuation of watchful waiting; a move upward of the PSA would signal the need to consider active intervention.

Furthermore, Dr. D'Amico stated in the December 2018 issue of *The New England Journal of Medicine* that, "This [Swedish] study proves that if a man is going to live 20–25 years and he's got prostate cancer, he has an opportunity to save his life."[7] As the NEJM article said, "that really means that men in the treatment [radical prostatectomy] group were able to live out their natural lives."

This outcome leads Dr. D'Amico to the conclusion that treatment is the preferable decision as opposed to active monitoring for healthy men age sixty-five or older.

CONSIDER THE BALANCE BETWEEN AGE AND TIME

Time horizons that are important to individual men will vary according to age. A young male will have a longer time horizon and, therefore, probably be more likely to risk the potential harms of screening in order to gain the potential benefits. However, he will have to live with harms, if they occur, for a longer period. The trade-off may not be as attractive for an older man with a shorter time horizon," according to the AUA guidelines, *Early Detection of Prostate Cancer.*[8]

In addition to the medical issues involved in the testing versus screening debate, other aspects merit examination, and they are the political and economic incentives.

The sequence of the following events is important:

- In 2008, USPSTF recommended against PSA screening for men older than seventy-five.
- Barack Obama's first term as president began on January 20, 2009.
- In 2009, the USPSTF became a political lightning rod for supporters of Obama's Affordable Care Act, and it began issuing opinions consistent with the politics of the day.
- In 2012, the task force "recommended against [screening] for all men, regardless of age, race, or family history."
- Obama's second term as president began on January 20, 2013.

- In November 2015, the federal government's Centers for Medicare & Medicaid Services (CMS), the operations manager for Medicare and Medicaid, proposed that doctors who order PSA screening tests should be financially penalized.
- Obama's second term of office ended on January 20, 2017.
- In late 2017, USPSTF modified its stand on PSA screening, stating that it would not discourage limited, cautious testing.

That CMS proposal was to have been included in new performance measures that it used to define quality care. Doctors who ordered PSA tests would contradict such performance measures under that proposal and would thus face financial consequences: doctors could be financially penalized for doing what they professionally believed was in the best interest of patients. CMS relented and dropped the proposal in March 2016; Obama left office on January 20, 2017.

In assessing the conflict, a 2017 Harvard prostate cancer report stated: "In 2012, the USPSTF gave PSA-based screening for prostate cancer a grade of D and recommended against routine testing for all men. The poor grade was based on evidence that only about one man in 1,000 who underwent screening would avoid death from prostate cancer. In fact, if a 55-year-old man chooses not to get screened, his chance of dying from prostate cancer over the next 10 to 15 years is about 0.6%. If he does choose to be screened, he reduces his chance of dying from the cancer to only 0.5%."[9]

"In 2012, if you were diagnosed with prostate cancer, you were almost certain to receive treatment. Now, the cancer is more likely to be observed," said Dr. Marc Garnick in 2017.[10] He is affiliated with Harvard's Beth Israel Deaconess Medical Center. He added, "The 15-year follow-up found little difference in death rates between men screened annually and those in the control group, who were screened occasionally. The researchers also noted that men with a PSA lower than 1.0 have only a 0.5% chance of being diagnosed with prostate cancer within 10 years."

IN OUR OPINION. . .

We conclude that a physician's decision regarding screening for prostate cancer, and how often a man should be screened, generally, are—and should be—influenced by four key elements:

1. *The medically demonstrated value of prostate screening*
2. *The desire to achieve as high a quality of life as possible for the patient*
3. *The potential harm that could result from a prostate cancer treatment that develops in the background (perhaps metastasizing)*
4. *Individual variables such as age, family history of prostate cancer, ethnicity, and dietary habits, among other considerations*

We further believe that the USPSTF has become a politically responsive organization that adopts or changes its position regarding its recommendations relative to prevailing political sentiment and potential economic implications as well as medical evidence.

A Dana-Farber/Harvard oncologist who regularly treats prostate cancer patients and survivors told us—as he put one hand over his eyes—"Not testing is like saying, 'I don't see it, so it isn't there.'"[11]

Regardless of the USPSTF's recommendations (which we believe are politically tainted), we as well as prostate cancer specialists stress the fact that the importance of an effective testing plan cannot be overstated. Indeed, the medical periodical UpToDate stated: "A screening program that could accurately identify asymptomatic men with aggressive localized tumors might be expected to substantially reduce prostate cancer morbidity, including urinary obstruction and painful metastases, and mortality.[12]

"Prostate cancer survival is related to many factors, especially the extent of [a] tumor at the time of diagnosis," the article continued, "The 5-year survival rate [for] men with cancer localized to the prostate or with only regional spread is 100%. This [success level] compares with a 29.3% survival rate among men with distant metastasized prostate cancer.[13]

CNN reported that researchers found that doctors could safely monitor a patient's prostate cancer—largely through repeated PSA checks—without rushing to treat it.

From our perspective, testing for prostate cancer is clearly related to quality-of-life issues. In order to avoid the painful—and sometimes debilitating—side effects of the various prostate cancer treatments, the cancer must be detected as early as possible—and before it metastasizes to other parts of the body. The earlier the diagnosis, and therefore stage of the disease, the less disabling will be the treatment's side effects. The least severe treatment is no treatment at all. Active surveillance aims to delay treatment until signs of progression are discovered, thus delaying the often permanent and unpleasant side effects of treatment until it's absolutely necessary.

The authors support screening to achieve early detection, which would permit less severe treatments than those characteristic of more advanced prostate cancers—especially those that have metastasized. Given that both age and the severity of a prostate cancer need to be considered in balance when deciding between active surveillance and treatment—rather than picking one over the other—we believe that the findings of a Dana-Farber radiation specialist are interesting.

Dr. Brandon Mahal led a Dana-Farber–Brigham and Women's Hospital study that indicated an increase in the cautious approach and showed an upsurge in active surveillance for low-risk prostate cancer.[14] *The conclusion of the five-year statistical study showed that, "Many men with low-risk prostate cancer, who most likely previously would have undergone immediate surgery or radiation, are now adopting a more conservative 'active surveillance' strategy," according to a February 2019 report on the study. Active surveillance "increased from 14.5 percent to 42.1 percent during the 2010–2015 study," while prostate gland removal (radical prostatectomy) declined from 47.4 percent to 31.3 percent. During the same period, the use of radiotherapy for low-risk disease dropped from 38.0 percent to 26.6 percent. "What we know from high level evidence is that conservative management of low-risk prostate cancer is associated with a very favorable prognosis," Dr. Mahal said. "Many men with low-risk disease are able to be spared the toxicity of treatment so it's an important discussion to have between clinicians and patients."*

Obviously, early detection and treatment can result in fewer and less severe side effects while preserving a higher quality of life with fewer psychological and physiological problems, including sexual impotence, urinary incontinence, and fecal incontinence.

6

Regular PSA Testing and Strategic Treatment

If you put your hands over your eyes and you don't see any evil, as one oncologist said, that doesn't mean that evil doesn't exist; it merely means that you may not see it.

That doctor suggested that his example dramatizes the conundrum faced by many prostate cancer patients when they are trying to decide if they want to be tested for the disease's presence. The fact that you don't know that prostate cancer is present in your body does not make it go away or cause it to be any less lethal. Yet, that is the conundrum faced by the government-sanctioned US Preventive Services Task Force.

It seems as though they want it both ways.

First, they said that all older men should be screened for prostate cancer. Then, because too many cases were detected and treated (sometimes inappropriately), they changed their stance, and stated that not testing was the right strategy. But, finally, they equivocated, and suggested that, well, maybe, strategic testing might be justified for certain individuals.

Such vacillating recommendations for a potentially devastating—even fatal—disease will leave many American men in a quandary: should they test and run the risk of a false positive, or not test and run the risk of developing an unstoppable metastatic cancer that will surely kill them if they live long enough.

Many cancer specialists believe that routine PSA testing, especially for men over the age of fifty, is highly desirable. Early detection, they believe, is critical to halting the spread of prostate cancer to other areas, often to the bones. This spreading of the cancer is called metastasizing, and if you don't die first of other causes, your metastatic prostate cancer will kill you.

One expert on and proponent of PSA testing, early detection, and strategic treatment is Dr. Anthony V. D'Amico,[1] who teaches at Harvard Medical School and is the head of the Division Chief of Genitourinary Radiation Oncology at the Dana-Farber Cancer Institute in Boston. Dr. D'Amico wrote in the October 13, 2016, issue of the *New England Journal of Medicine*: "For today, we can conclude . . . that PSA monitoring, as compared with treatment of early prostate cancer, leads to increased metastasis. Therefore, if a man wishes to avoid metastatic prostate cancer and the side effects of its treatment, monitoring should be considered only if he has [a] life-threatening disease such that his life expectancy is less than 10-year[s]."[2]

Let's parse Dr. D'Amico's statement into simple sentences, and then take the long view:

1. PSA monitoring "leads to increased metastasis."
2. To "avoid metastatic prostate cancer," a man should choose an alternative to mere PSA monitoring.
3. A man should choose PSA monitoring only if he expects to die of other causes within ten years.

We believe, however, that before a man makes such a dramatic decision, he should also take into consideration three statements made by the Social Security Administration (SSA), which says:

- A man reaching age sixty-five today can expect to live on until age eighty-four.[3]
- 25 percent of sixty-five-year-olds will live past age ninety.
- 10 percent of sixty-five-year-olds will live past age ninety-five.

Stated yet another way: If you do not expect to die within the next ten years, you should check to see if you have an elevated PSA. Thus, the Social Security Administration's (SSA) life projections put a whole new light on:

- The phrase "Ten years or less to live"
- The very real issue of quality of life
- Whether to stop PSA testing at age seventy

Based on the three SSA statistical statements, a man would *not* stop testing—expecting to live another ten years—until between the ages of seventy-four and eighty-five. Therefore, we believe that many men would find choosing watchful waiting for overactive PSA test results to be an unacceptable option. Similarly, Dr. D'Amico would choose the "regular PSA testing" path because it allows for early detection and rapid and strategic treatment. Why is this so? The obvious answer is "metastases," which means that the cancer cells that developed in the prostate break free of that organ and begin to circulate in a man's body. Once free, these cancer cells can establish separate areas of growth in other tissues elsewhere in the body. Therefore, without treatment, the prostate cancer cells are allowed time to metastasize (or spread) to other locations.

What Are Lymph Nodes?

Lymph nodes, also referred to as lymph glands, are an important part of the immune system. They are located throughout the body but are visible and palpable only when they are enlarged or swollen.

Lymph nodes are regional, and each group of them corresponds to a particular region of the body and reflects abnormalities in that region.

Common areas where swollen lymph nodes are more prominent and therefore more readily noticeable are behind the ear, in the neck, the chin, the armpits, and in the groin.

Doctors and other healthcare professionals also check these areas for enlarged or swollen lymph nodes. Lymph is a watery fluid that circulates within the lymphatic vessels. Lymph nodes are found near these vessels.

Within the capsule, lymph nodes contain certain kinds of immune cells. These cells are mainly lymphocytes, which produce proteins that capture and fight viruses and other microbes.

A favorite location of prostate cancer cells is a man's bones. If that happens, the area of bony metastasis is still prostate cancer—not bone cancer—even though it is located in your bones.

Prostate cancer metastasis means "the cancer cells travel through the lymphatic system or the bloodstream to other areas of the body,"[3] according to Dr. Erik P. Castle, an associate professor of urology at the College of Medicine at the Mayo Clinic. The lymph nodes are a key part of the immune system and contain a dense collection of lymphocytes, which are a type of white blood cell. "Commonly, prostate cancer metastasis can occur in the bones, lymph nodes, lung, liver or brain." However, "it's rarer for it to move to . . . the brain," says *Web*MD.[4] Patients with such bony metastases will need therapy for the rest of their lives, which could include radiation, chemotherapy, and Androgen Deprivation Therapy.

In considering your options, you should know that metastatic prostate cancer is considered an advanced form of cancer, for which there is no cure. *You can treat metastatic prostate cancer, but you cannot cure it.* Dr. D'Amico is clear in his *New England Journal of Medicine* article: "The clinical significance . . . is that with the use of active monitoring [without testing], more men will have metastasis . . . which is not insignificant." "Not insignificant," indeed! While you don't want prostate cancer, you really don't want metastatic prostate cancer!

Healthline.com states that the changes in a man's life that accompany metastatic cancer include:

- Bone pain
- Weak bones, increasing your risk for fractures
- Spinal cord compression and related weakness or numbness
- High blood calcium levels
- Stiffness or pain in the hip, thighs, or back

"These symptoms can cause severe discomfort and disability. Spinal cord compression can result in nerve damage, which can lead to muscle weakness or paralysis, numbness in the legs or arms, or loss of control of bladder and bowel functions," according to Healthline.com, which also notes that "higher levels of calcium in the blood can occur as cancer replaces normal bone," triggering vomiting, dehydration, confusion, and abdominal discomfort.[5]

Despite the significantly diminished quality of life associated with metastatic prostate cancer, contrarians continue to take a dim view of regular PSA testing. Those adherents believe such routine screening can lead to overtreatment, which creates its own set of quality-of-life problems and generates potentially needless costs that generally are paid by insurance companies.

If one believes that the average lifespan of white men in the United States is 76.3 years and neglects those men living into their eighties or nineties, then the watchful-waiting approach makes perfect sense and eliminates the need for annual or semiannual insurance-paid PSA-related tests and the possible additional expenses of surgery, radiation, and chemical/hormone therapy.[6] The watchful-waiting approach, however, does not take into account the human misery that comes when a prostate cancer metastasizes to other parts of the body.

Nonetheless, the U.S. Preventive Services Task Force (USPSTF) has broadly recommended against PSA screening for prostate cancer:[7] "The main goal of annual PSA cancer screening test is to reduce the number of deaths from the disease. The Task Force found that among adult men, only a very small number, if any, would experience this benefit as a result of screening" when compared to a monitoring approach, or watchful waiting.[8]

Our question to the task force is: *"Who among you wants to be in that 'very small number' of men who may suffer, or even die, from metastatic prostate cancer because you did not have a PSA test?"*

Nonetheless, the task force reinforces its argument against regular prostate screening based on the potential harms found as a result of PSA screening.

The [annual] PSA screening test often suggests that prostate cancer may be present when there is no cancer. This is called a "false-positive" result. False-positive results cause worry and anxiety and can lead to follow-up tests that aren't needed. . . . If prostate cancer is diagnosed, there is no way currently to tell for sure if it is a cancer that will never cause a problem and does not need treatment or if it is an aggressive cancer that does need treatment. This means that many non-harmful cancers are diagnosed. This is called "over-diagnosis."

Let us refer back to Dr. D'Amico's NEJM article: "For today, we can conclude . . . that PSA monitoring—as compared with treatment of early prostate cancer—leads to increased metastasis. Therefore, if a man wishes to avoid metastatic prostate cancer and the side effects of its treatment, monitoring should be considered only if he has [another] life-threatening disease [that makes it likely] his life expectancy is less than the 10-year median."

We agree, therefore, that the USPSTF's numbers-based conclusion

- Is conservative (at best).
- Does not consider quality-of-life issues.
- Clearly does not take into account the SSA's statistics that many men will live well into their eighties and nineties.

Not performing annual PSA tests for prostate cancer is like throwing men under the bus. Indeed, a man's longevity and quality of life must be considered in tandem. If a man misses the "window of beneficial treatment," as one doctor described it, that miss could have severe implications for years to come.

Despite the recalcitrance of the USPSTF, insurance companies generally cover annual PSA tests for men over fifty, as does Medicare. While the American Cancer Society "supports legislation assuring that men have insurance coverage for prostate screening exams," it concedes that there exist differing opinions about the value of screening in an effort to "lower the risk of dying from prostate cancer." [9] It qualifies its position with the statement that it "does not recommend routine testing for prostate cancer for all men at this time . . . [and that] doctors and other health care providers should offer information on the potential risks and benefits of prostate-specific antigen testing to appropriate patients, allowing them to make an informed decision on testing." This position seems to be a form of "passing the buck" of responsibility regarding the decision to test or not to test. In other words, you can't point a finger at the ACS and blame them.

Nonetheless, state legislatures, largely populated by men, seem to have risen to the occasion and enacted laws on a variety of prostate cancer issues, including:

- Assured health insurance coverage for prostate cancer screening
- Public education on prostate cancer
- Prostate cancer research funds

It seems that while there may be equivocation among some institutions, one ACS report acknowledges that, "Many states have laws assuring that private health insurers cover tests to detect prostate cancer, including the PSA test and DRE."[10] Some states also ensure that public employee benefit health plans provide coverage for prostate cancer screening tests. Most state laws ensure annual coverage for men fifty and over and for high-risk men beginning at age forty. High risk refers to African American men and men with a family history of prostate cancer. Some states have slightly different coverage requirements.[11]

Having made our case for prostate cancer testing, we must add the recent research results that were published in the June 2019 Harvard Health Letter.[12] It wrote: "New findings show a dramatic increase in the number of men taking a conservative approach to low-risk prostate cancer." The records of 165,000 men show that the level of "active surveillance" tripled from 2010 to 2015. Among men with "low-risk prostate cancer," active surveillance increased from 15 percent to 42 percent from 2010 to 2015. During the same period, surgery fell from 47 percent to 31 percent, and radiation treatment dropped from 38 percent to 27 percent. Nonetheless, we still favor regular, cautious prostate cancer testing.

IN OUR OPINION. . .

Despite the fact that the USPSTF, a federal organization responsible for making medical treatment recommendations, has wavered considerably (we have written about this vacillation in depth elsewhere in this book) on the value of testing for prostate cancer, or not, we unquestionably believe that early, regular, and careful testing is the gold standard for detection of the disease.

We must emphasize that when prostate cancer is detected in its early stages, before it has metastasized, the chances of curing the disease are nearly 100 percent. If the disease spreads to other parts of the body, however, the chances of a man's survival are considerably reduced.

As the cliché goes, "better safe than sorry." However, we do believe that there is an opportunity to overreact to test results, and that is why we believe that early, regular testing should be accompanied with an abundance of professional caution. That said, you do not want to miss a prostate cancer that is real, and that could metastasize and possibly take your life.

7

Testing and Your Quality of Life

Determining your desired quality of life is neither a simple exercise nor one that a person regularly undertakes. Indeed, "quality of life" is often something that just happens, merely a result of other decisions we make about our lives, family demands, and what jobs we pursue. Each of those has a significant impact on the quality our lives, as well as the lives of our partners and spouses.

Probably the one life-changing event that you likely have given very little thought to, until now, is prostate cancer and its treatment. Not only have you previously given little thought to the disease, but you likely have given even less thought to the potential impact prostate cancer will have on the lives of those closest to you, especially your partner or spouse.

We are fairly certain that most men, once they're aware of that impact, will take prostate cancer seriously. However, many of them don't think sufficiently about the quality of life they can expect as they live through the challenges of prostate cancer.

Note that we did not say, "Pass through this challenge called prostate cancer," because you pass into it, not through it. And that is a very important fact to come to grips with. Frankly, we believe that there should never be a question of "Do I or don't I" receive treatment for your disease.

The only real questions are: "How soon should I begin treatment?" and "Which treatments should I undergo?" Ideally, these decisions should be made in consultation with your oncologists, with the insightful assistance of a professional prostate counselor, also known as a personal decision assistant, and your partner or spouse. (The subject of "Managing My Prostate Cancer Decisions" is discussed later in this book.)

When you are in the middle of a fight—as with prostate cancer—it may not be the best time to make delicate, difficult decisions. However, it is the only opportunity you have.

Richard Hoffman, a professor of internal medicine and epidemiology at the University of Iowa's Carver College of Medicine in Iowa City, set out to learn if prostate cancer patients have regretted their treatment decisions. Hoffman's team sampled 934 men at one, two, five, and fifteen years after they had been diagnosed with prostate cancer in the 1990s. Each survey participant was seventy-five or younger when he was diagnosed with tumors confined to the prostate itself, that is, the cancer had not spread or metastasized. "Most of the men (89%) were treated with surgery or radiation. The rest were lumped together as having had conservative treatment: either medications to suppress testosterone . . . or 'watchful waiting,'" according to Harvard Health Publishing, which summarized the research. The findings showed that 14.6 percent of the entire group expressed some treatment regret, and among the causes of regret, treatment-related bowel and sexual problems were cited most frequently. Surgically treated men, 15 percent of the whole group, reported the highest rate of regret, 39 percent, of significant sexual side effects. About 16 percent of radiation-treated men complained about significant bowl problems.

The medical newsletter *STAT* wrote about that Iowa study and reported that, "after years of introspection, a small percentage of the [nearly] 1,000 patients with localized prostate cancer had regrets about their decisions regarding treatment."[1] (We don't consider 14, 15, and 16 percent as small percentages.) This could result from some individuals having received inadequate counseling, or the patient's failure to recognize the significance of the treatment outcome.

We also believe that the unfortunate fact is that many times, it is virtually impossible to adequately convey to a patient the full impact prostate cancer treatment will have on his body, mind, and spirit—and that he will likely endure these changes.

Problems that caused regret were:

- Treated surgically, 39 percent reported significant sexual side effects.
- Treated with radiation, 15.6 percent reported significant bowl problems; 17.6 percent reported urinary incontinence.

- Treated with the more conservative method of watchful waiting, 15.5 percent complained of urinary incontinence.

STAT also reported, "Results also showed that regret tends to increase with time, suggesting that when initial concerns over surviving prostate cancer wear off, the quality-of-life consequences of treatment become more apparent," and that, not surprisingly, "Regrets were especially pronounced among men who felt they hadn't been sufficiently counseled by their doctors" before selecting a treatment option, and "among men who were preoccupied with changing levels of Prostate-Specific Antigen."

These results again indicate that inadequate counseling and education often take place before prostate cancer patients select and undergo a course of treatment.

The *Journal of Clinical Oncology* concluded in a July 2017 article:

"Regret was a relatively infrequently reported outcome among long-term survivors of localized prostate cancer; however, our results suggest that better informing men about treatment options, in particular, conservative treatment, might help mitigate long-term regret. These findings are timely for men with low-risk cancers who are being encouraged to consider active surveillance."[2]

The Cancer Treatment Centers of America (CTCA) emphasized the need for real world caution as the institution related on its website, CancerCenter.com; when Mark P. was diagnosed with prostate cancer in 2014, he "was in complete shock."[3] He explains his actions on the CTCA website.

I took my time deciding on a course of action. Even though the diagnosis was clear. . . . When I heard that I might need six to eight weeks of radiation treatment, I became overwhelmed. . . . Right away, there were people (at CTCA) giving me not only medical attention but whole-person attention.

By September 2015, it was time to take action. I chose to have a prostatectomy to surgically remove the cancer. . . . I wasn't prepared for the aftermath of a prostatectomy.

Today (January 2017), I am still recovering from the surgery and am continuing to make progress. My PSA score indicates minor residual cancer, so my oncologist is continuing to monitor me. I have regained nearly all my normal functions.[4]

USE OF MRI IN DEALING WITH PROSTATE CANCER[5]

Increased PSA screening may have resulted in fewer cancer-related deaths in recent years, but it also *increased detection* of prostate cancer and *unnecessary treatment*. In some cases, that treatment could have been of men who would have died from other causes before their prostate cancer metastasized and killed them.

However, the use of Magnetic Resonance Imaging (MRI) has begun to change the test-or-not conundrum: test and run the risk of unnecessary treatment, or don't test and run the risk of metastatic cancer. Major technical improvements in the MRI process have resulted in its expanded role in prostate cancer management. The areas of currently recognized value of MRI in treating prostate cancer includes the following situations:

- If a prostate biopsy is strongly indicated—but results are negative—further MRI imaging is the most valid and accepted technique.
- If there is a likelihood that a pre-biopsy MRI would improve the diagnosis of the disease.
- If a prostate MRI would aid in the staging.
- If MRIs can augment or replace follow-up biopsies in men on active surveillance to ensure that high-grade cancer has is not missed.
- If radiation therapy for localized prostate cancer is not successful, or for being considered for salvage prostatectomy.

Most men with prostate cancer in the United States receive surgery or radiation to treat their prostate cancer. If a residual cancer exists or disease recurs after one of these treatments, it can be treated with a salvage prostatectomy,[6] a procedure performed after radiation treatment has failed, according to University of California San Francisco Health.

TESTING, TREATING, AND WAITING: A COMPLEX DECISION

Any quality-of-life assessment for men who are being treated for prostate cancer is complex. Simply stated, any radiation or surgical treatment leads to partial or total erectile dysfunction and urinary or fecal incontinence, and these consequences may be lifelong.

No screening test is perfect. Some tests like the DRE (digital rectal exam) are not very sensitive and will miss many early prostate cancers. Other tests, like the PSA test can generate a significant number of false positive results.

Prostate biopsies and treatments targeting localized prostate cancer carry risks, the AUA warns. "For every 1,000 men tested, approximately 10% to 12% will have an elevated PSA. Among those diagnosed with prostate cancer, about 90% will undergo treatment,"[7] it says. The men treated will experience one of three outcomes:

1. No evidence of prostate cancer because their disease was in error.
2. Recurrent cancer that will progress despite their treatment.
3. Neither evidence of prostate cancer recurrence nor any benefit from treatment because their cancer was never destined to progress.

The AUA also says, "For every 1,000 men who are screened for prostate cancer,

- 2 will develop serious cardiovascular events.
- 1 will develop deep venous thrombosis (blood clot) or pulmonary embolus (blockage).
- 29 will develop erectile dysfunction.
- 18 will develop incontinence.
- Less than 1% (fewer than 10) will die from treatment."[8]

Estimates from the European trial (ERSPC) indicate the following outcomes:

- ~ sixty men of every one thousand between the ages of fifty-five and sixty-nine will develop clinical evidence of prostate cancer within ten to fourteen years if they choose *not* to be screened, and five will die of their disease within ten to fourteen years.

- ~ ninety-six men of every one thousand will be diagnosed with prostate cancer if they choose to be screened, and four will die of their disease within ten to fourteen years.

Watchful waiting, however, can create an observation period during which a man would be free of those complications and thus ensure a better quality of life, at least for a time.

The trade-off between observation (watchful waiting) and treatment, however, is the increased risk of metastatic prostate cancer. As we have written earlier, even if the prostate cancer spreads, or metastasizes, to the bones or elsewhere in the body, it remains "prostate cancer," regardless of its physical location.

If it metastasizes, one would be subjected to a lifelong treatment program that would likely include Androgen Deprivation Therapy (ADT). This results in complications that include erectile dysfunction and the onset of one or both forms of incontinence, urinary and fecal.

In addition to the problems noted above, the side effects of ADT are very unpleasant and include reduced sexual desire, fatigue, muscle-wasting and consequent weakness, and lack of endurance and of enthusiasm, as well as specific physiological changes, including loss of body hair, breast enlargement, shrinkage of the penis and testicles, and hot flashes.

If a man selects observation and is lucky, his prostate cancer will develop slowly, which will allow him to avoid ADT and its quite unpleasant side effects during his lifetime.

A DIFFERENT SET OF OUTCOMES

The results of a study of 1,201 patients and 625 spouses or partners by Emory University's Dr. Martin G. Sanda provide a less-confident outcome. His team sought to identify the factors among patients that influenced their opinions about quality of life. Thus, in making this determination, it is important to understand the relationship between 1) what you consider personally important in life and 2) your attitude about the quality of life overall. The team believed that assessing how those quality-of-life determinants might change as a result of treatment would help them understand why patients' quality-of-life perspectives also change.

(Dr. Sanda is a prostate cancer surgeon and scientist, chair of the Department of Urology at Emory, and director of the Prostate Cancer Center at the school's Winship Cancer Institute. He previously taught urology at Harvard Medical School and practiced medicine at Beth Israel Deaconess and Dana-Farber Cancer Center in Boston.)

Broadly stated, the team found that, "Each prostate-cancer treatment was associated with a distinct pattern of change in Quality-of-Life" that related to urinary, sexual, bowel, and hormonal function. Not surprisingly, "These changes influenced satisfaction with treatment outcomes among patients and their spouses or partners."[9]

Adjuvant (auxiliary) hormone therapy was associated with worse outcomes across multiple quality-of-life domains among patients receiving brachytherapy or radiotherapy. With the brachytherapy (seed implantation) or radiotherapy group, patients reported having long-lasting urinary irritation, bowel and sexual symptoms, and transient problems with vitality or hormonal function. With the prostatectomy group, patients reported urinary incontinence, but their urinary irritation and obstruction improved, particularly in patients with large prostates. Patients reported that nerve-sparing procedures lessened adverse effects on sexual function. No treatment-related deaths occurred, and serious adverse events were rare. The team reported that the "treatment-related symptoms were exacerbated by obesity, a large prostate size, a high PSA score, and older age." Black patients were less satisfied with overall treatment outcomes.

IN OUR OPINION. . .

The seriousness of prostate cancer cannot be overstated, although it often is dismissed with the platitude that, "Oh well, you know that men die with prostate cancer, not of it."

Because prostate cancer can be a life-or-death issue, we believe that a good amount of reading, inquiry, counseling, and thought will help ensure fewer surprises and better outcomes. It is not uncommon, in our experience, to have a fully competent oncology team touch all the bases—surgery, hormone, radiation, and their aftereffects—and still not have a single medical professional suggest contacting a counselor or provide you with an introduction to one.

Indeed, we believe, that no oncology team is complete without an experienced prostate cancer counselor, who will explain the "real world" implications of the doctors' procedures, their impact on your personal life and psychology, as well as the impact each can have on your spouse.

Unfortunately, this fourth wheel on the cancer team vehicle is often missing, and that is to the disadvantage of the patient. You will have enough problems dealing with your disease; don't make matters worse by keeping yourself in the dark. It may be a cliché, but the fact is that "knowledge is power," and we're in favor of empowering you with all of the knowledge you can get—and handle.

8

What Are the Tests, and What Do They Mean?

Having a prostate-specific antigen (PSA) test is just the beginning. It is a laboratory test that—when the results are elevated—implies that you might have some degree of prostate cancer. Further tests may confirm that indication. While elevated PSA test results may indicate the presence of prostate cancer, however, they also may indicate other conditions that are less serious.

The PSA test is performed as the first step of your blood test workup, and it could have a significant impact on your quality of life. It is not something to take lightly; it is not "just another test," and what it indicates could change the remainder for your life—physically and psychologically—as well as your interpersonal relationships.

This chapter will help you understand the sequence of tests that your personal or family doctor and oncologist may order to help define the nature of your prostate cancer. Determining the extent to which your cancer has invaded your body will help your doctor determine the best strategies for treating it.

The American Urological Association (AUA) warns about the gravity of the possible consequences of the prostate cancer screening process. The AUA states that while only some men benefit from prostate cancer treatment, all men who are treated are "exposed to the complications of treatment," and it believes that before making a decision about prostate testing or screening, a man needs to know a specific set of facts,[1] that will materially influence his decisions regarding whether to proceed with testing, then, if needed, his treatment selection. Regarding the statistics that follow, the AUA cautions that, "these are estimates *for men deciding on screening*, not men who are deciding on treatment *after diagnosis*."

While many men are diagnosed with prostate cancer, "only a minority [3%] will ever progress to the point where the disease is considered advanced and even fewer will have a fatal prostate cancer."[2] Therefore, "men should consider the threat posed by prostate cancer and weigh this against other potential life-threatening conditions." Read another way, that statement simply means: The older you are, the more likely you are to die of another cause during the next ten years—therefore, prostate cancer screening is less important for you.

The AUA states that these results amount to "one life saved by screening for every 1,000 men; however, models have projected that over a man's lifetime, the number of lives saved by screening could be as many as 6 per 1,000 men screened.[3, 4]

Now, let's move on to the specific tests that you may encounter and what they are all about.

THE PROSTATE-SPECIFIC ANTIGEN BLOOD TEST

As you know from reading previous chapters of this book, the PSA test is controversial, and a moving target. For instance, the USPSTF first recommended widespread PSA testing, then changed and recommended against it, and now recommends limited and cautious testing.

The PSA blood test is often performed as part of a man's annual physical exam—especially when he is over fifty—and is used mainly to screen for evidence of prostate cancer in men without symptoms. It is also one of the first tests done in men who *do* have prostate cancer symptoms.

The PSA test determines the amount of prostate-specific antigen present in a man's blood. Both cancerous as well as noncancerous tissues in the prostate produce the PSA protein. If the level of PSA increases above a normal level, it *may indicate* prostate cancer; however, other factors can cause an elevated PSA, including inflammation. And what is considered "normal" may vary by half a point from institution to institution; Johns Hopkins is a bit more conservative in how it uses the text than Mayo Clinic Labs, for instance.[5, 6]

As stated earlier, the PSA blood test is the first step in the screening process. If your PSA score concerns your physician, he likely will schedule a second test in a few weeks; if he is more concerned, he will schedule a biopsy to further assess the condition of your prostate. The biopsy results are then graded by the testing pathologist using one of two, or possibly both, prostate cancer grading systems.

When prostate cancer is detected, your physician will assign your case to one of three "risk groups"—low, medium, or high—which is determined by results from:

1. Your PSA test
2. Your digital rectal exam (DRE) results
3. Your biopsy

The numbers below are provided by *Men's Hormonal Health* (*MHH*) and can be used as a broad outline of "normal PSA levels" for Asian, African American, and Caucasian men.[7]

Table 8.1. Normal PSA Levels

Age	Asian	African	Caucasian
40–49	0–2.0 ng/ml	0–2.0 ng/ml	0–2.5 ng/ml
50–59	0–3.0 ng/ml	0–4.0 ng/ml	0–3.5 ng/ml
60–69	0–4.0 ng/ml	0–4.5 ng/ml	0–4.5 ng/ml
70–79	0–5.0 ng/ml	0–5.5 ng/ml	0–6.5 ng/ml

MHH cautions that, "Higher standards are necessary but [are] not sufficient proof that PSA testing will reduce mortality from prostate cancer. . . . Studies of PSA density have reported mixed findings." Therefore, the guidance of your own urologist should provide you with insight into your particular case. That said, *MMH* provides the following guidelines and steps for categorizing PSA levels.

Table 8.2. PSA Level Categories

Normal PSA	0 – 4 ng/ml
Slightly Elevated PSA	4 – 10 ng/ml
Moderately Elevated PSA	10 – 20 ng/ml
Highly Elevated PSA	20 + ng/ml

ADDITIONAL TESTS AND NEXT STEPS

The Gleason Score[8]

Gleason scores range from between 2 and 10, and they grade the prostate according to how "normal" it appears. A grade of 1 means the prostate looks normal; however, the American Cancer Society says that a Gleason score of 1 and 2 is seldom used because most prostates achieve a grade of 3 or higher. Most Gleason scores are 6 through 10. The higher your Gleason score, the more likely it is your cancer will grow and spread quickly.

- Gleason 6 or less: well-differentiated, low-grade
- Gleason 7: moderately differentiated, intermediate-grade
- Gleason 8, 9, or 10: poorly differentiated, high-grade

Physicians think about localized or locally advanced prostate cancer in terms of "risk groups," which are assigned before the patient undergoes any treatment. There are three general risk groups based on the PSA, DRE, and biopsy, which can be further subdivided to better personalize one's treatment.

- Low risk: Tumor confined to the prostate; Gleason score of 6 or lower.
- Intermediate risk: Tumor confined to the prostate; Gleason score of 7. This category is often divided into a "favorable" and "unfavorable" intermediate risk.
- High risk: Tumor extends outside the prostate, PSA Gleason score of 8, 9, or 10. There is also a subset of very aggressive tumors called "very high risk" in which the tumor has extended into the seminal vesicles.

The treatment options for each risk group are quite different, and you should ask your doctor which risk group you belong to so you can better understand the most appropriate next steps.

Biopsy

If your PSA level is 3 or 4, your doctor is likely to recommend a biopsy, but that does not necessarily mean you have prostate cancer. That's why a biopsy is performed, to see if there is cause for concern, or not. Indeed, there may be no cancer found, but some cancers may be present even at this low or even lower PSA levels. It all depends on each individual's unique characteristics and progression of the disease.

The two most common forms of biopsy are the Transrectal Ultrasound–guided (TRUS) biopsy and the transperineal biopsy.

Transrectal Ultrasound, or TRUS

The transrectal ultrasound procedure is used to generate sound waves, which create images of your prostate. This is about a ten-minute outpatient examination and is usually performed in a doctor's office. During the procedure, a finger-sized probe is inserted into your rectum; it emits sound waves, which are then translated into images of your prostate. "Your doctor will use the images to identify the area that needs to be numbed with an injection to reduce discomfort associated with the biopsy. The ultrasound images are also used to guide the prostate biopsy needle into place," according to the Mayo Clinic.[9]

During the actual biopsy procedure, your doctor will retrieve thin, cylindrical sections of tissue with a spring-propelled needle. The procedure typically causes a very brief uncomfortable sensation each time the spring-loaded needle takes a sample. Generally, your doctor will take ten to twelve tissue samples during the procedure, which takes about ten minutes. The sample of tissue that is removed from the prostate is then examined under a microscope. "The problem with ultrasound is that it cannot easily distinguish cancerous tissue from healthy tissue," says New York's Dr. Samadi. "In fact, needles guided by transrectal ultrasound miss potentially aggressive high-grade tumors a full 40 percent of the time."

"Biomedical engineers have addressed this deficiency by adding high-resolution pictures of the prostate made by a newer technology called multi-parametric magnetic resonance imaging (MP-MRI) into the mix. Prostate tumors show up on MP-MRI as dark spots, and by adding MP-MRI images taken beforehand to the real-time ultrasound images, urologists can target suspicious regions of the gland while steering clear of healthy tissue. Engineers call this enhanced-tech procedure a 'fusion-guided biopsy.'"

Transperineal Biopsy

The main benefit of the transperineal biopsy is safety, according to the Mayo Clinic. This is due to the lower risk of severe infection. They also say that "with a transperineal approach, it is much easier to access the anterior [foremost part of the] prostate, which is not well sampled with transrectal biopsy." In a transperineal biopsy, a needle is placed into the prostate and "there are several different techniques by which we can perform transperineal biopsy," according to Mayo's Dr. Derek J. Lomas. The choice of technique is based on whether a fusion or a systematic biopsy is needed and if the patient is in the clinic or under sedation. A transperineal biopsy is fine for all patients, according to Mayo, especially those with a:

• History of infection after a previous transrectal biopsy
• History of prostatitis
• Inflammatory bowel disease
• Rectal bleeding complications after a previous biopsy
• Previous negative transrectal biopsy with suspicion of anterior prostate tumor

Bone Scan

This procedure is used to determine if your prostate cancer has metastasized to the bone, which usually is the first target when cancer spreads to distant parts of your body. The test involves injecting you with a low-level radioactive material, which is most readily absorbed by areas of cancer in affected bones.

"A bone scan may suggest cancer in the bone," The ACS writes, "but to make an accurate diagnosis, other tests such as plain X-rays, CT or MRI scans, or even a bone biopsy might be needed."

Computerized Tomography, or CT or CAT Scan

Almost always an outpatient procedure, a CT scan takes up to thirty minutes and can show your doctor the size and shape of your cancer tumor. The scan uses x-rays to make a detailed, cross-sectional body image and can help determine if your prostate cancer has spread into nearby lymph nodes. If you have already been treated for prostate cancer, and it appears to have returned, a CT scan may be able to determine if your cancer has extended into other organs or parts of your body.

This test isn't often needed for newly diagnosed prostate cancer if your doctor has decided that the cancer is likely to be confined to the prostate. Such a conclusion is based on other findings that include your DRE results, PSA level, and Gleason score.

Doctors may use a CT scan in a procedure called a CT-guided biopsy. This image helps them accurately insert a needle to remove a tissue sample. "CT scans can also be used to guide needles into tumors for some types of cancer treatments, such as radio frequency ablation (RFA), which uses heat to destroy a tumor," according to the American Cancer Society. Comparing multiple CT scans taken over time allows doctors to determine how a tumor is responding to treatment or if a cancer has returned after treatment.

Magnetic Resonance Imaging, or MRI

Like CT scans, Magnetic Resonance Imaging (MRI) scans show detailed images of soft tissues in the body, but MRI scans use radio waves and strong magnets instead of X-rays. A contrast material called gadolinium may be injected into a vein before the scan to better see details.

MRI scans can give a very clear picture of the prostate and show if the cancer has spread outside the prostate into the seminal vesicles (which "produce and store fluid that will eventually become semen") or other nearby structures.[10] This can be very important in determining your treatment options, but like CT scans, MRI scans aren't usually needed for newly diagnosed cancers that are likely to be confined to the prostate based on other factors.

To improve the accuracy of the MRI, you might have a probe, called an endorectal coil, placed inside your rectum for the scan. This can be uncomfortable. If needed, medicine to make you feel sleepy while relaxing the anal muscles can be given before the scan.

Lymph Node Biopsy

A lymph node biopsy, sometimes called a lymphadenectomy, is not a common procedure with prostate cancer; however, it may be done to determine if your cancer has spread to the lymph nodes. The procedure involves removing one or more lymph nodes to look for cancer cells.

Lymph nodes are discussed elsewhere in this book, but here is further information on them: "Lymph nodes are small, bean-shaped organs which produce and store a type of white blood cells (lymphocytes) that help fight disease and infection. Also known as lymph glands, lymph nodes remove cell waste and fluids from lymph (lymphatic fluid). Lymph nodes are part of the lymphatic system and are located throughout the body, including the neck, armpits, abdomen and groin," according to Cancer Treatment Centers of America. "Lymph nodes play an important role in cancer staging, which determines the extent of cancer in the body."

Lymph Node Biopsy During Surgery

Lymph nodes in the pelvis may be removed during a radical prostatectomy if your surgeon believes that there is more than a very small chance that your cancer may have spread outside the prostate. "More often (especially if the chance of cancer spread is low), the lymph nodes and the prostate are removed and are then sent to the lab" to be examined,[11] according to ACS.

While a lymph node biopsy is seldom performed as a separate procedure from prostate surgery, the procedure may be undertaken when a radical prostatectomy is not anticipated but your doctor still wants to know if your cancer has invaded the lymph nodes.

Staging of Prostate Cancer

While there are multiple staging systems, one of the most common ones is the TNM method, which indicates how far the cancer has progressed. In this method, the extent of the tumor is represented by T, the extent of disease's spread to the lymph nodes is represented by N, and the extent to which the cancer has spread, or metastasized, is represented by M.

"If there's no cancer found in the lymph nodes near the cancer, the N is assigned a value of 0. If nearby or distant nodes show cancer, the N is assigned a number (such as 1, 2, or 3), depending on how many nodes are affected, how much cancer is in them, how large they are, and where they are."[12]

Your surgeon may remove lymph nodes in the pelvis during the same operation as the removal of the prostate, which is known as a radical prostatectomy. If there is more than a very small chance that the cancer might have spread (based on factors such as a high PSA level or a high Gleason score), the surgeon may remove some lymph nodes before removing the prostate gland.

Sometimes, the nodes will be examined right away, while you are still under anesthesia, to help the surgeon decide whether to continue with the radical prostatectomy. This is called a frozen section exam because the tissue sample is frozen before thin slices are taken to check under a microscope. If the nodes contain cancer cells, the operation might be stopped (leaving the prostate in place). This could happen if the surgeon feels that removing the prostate would be unlikely to cure the cancer but would probably result in undesirable complications or side effects.

More often (especially if the chance of cancer spread is low), a frozen section exam is not done. Instead, the lymph nodes and the prostate are removed and are then sent to the lab to be examined. The lab results are usually available several days after surgery. "A man's prognosis depends on the stage of the cancer when it is diagnosed," according to the 2019 *Annual Report on Prostate Cancer*, published by the Harvard Medical School.[13] If the cancer is confined to the prostate when it is detected, "the five-year prostate cancer-specific survival rate is nearly 100%," according to the Harvard report. If, however, the cancer has spread to the "lymph nodes, bone or other organ when it is diagnosed, the five-year survival rate is substantially lower."[14]

Cascade Testing

Cascade genetic testing is different from PSA screening because it helps determine "whether family members share a genetic mutation."[15] While a positive test is not conclusive evidence of inherited prostate cancer, it does put that individual at "increased risk." The power of genetic testing to aid in cancer prevention is amplified with cascade testing.

Cascade testing helps identify your hereditary linkage with cancer. Genetic counselors help identify family members with the same genetic mutation as the patient. "Most, but not all, of the genetic mutations related to hereditary cancer are passed down at a rate of 50%," according to the University of Texas's Southwestern Medical Center in Dallas.[16]

"Having a genetic mutation does not mean the individual will definitely develop cancer," the university states. "It simply indicates an increased risk. . . . Inherited risk for prostate cancer is associated with [an] aggressive disease and poorer outcomes, indicating a critical need for increased genetic screening to more accurately identify individuals at increased risk for metastatic castration-resistant cancer," according to Piper Nicolas, PhD at Invitae Corp. in San Francisco.[17]

Dr. Nicolas' comment came in response to a February 2019 article in the *Journal of the American Medical Association* that stated, "Results from a recent cross-sectional study suggest that National Comprehensive Cancer Network guidelines and Gleason scores are not reliable for stratifying patients with prostate cancer." It further suggested that expanding those guidelines "will improve medical management of those [prostate cancer] patients."

On yet another front, female family members who test positive also may be at risk for other cancers such as breast, pancreatic, ovarian, and gastrointestinal cancers.

Postsurgery PSA

PSA testing after surgery or radiation therapy is not an exact science and may include a urologist, oncologist, and others. Although a high PSA may increase a doctor's suspicion of prostate cancer, an elevated PSA alone does not confirm a diagnosis of prostate cancer. An elevated PSA may also be caused by trauma, infection, and other noncancerous conditions. Surgery, radiation therapy, and/or Androgen Deprivation Therapy do not eliminate all PSA, but their levels are substantially reduced.

Measuring and using PSA velocity (which changes over time) is an art, not a science. There is no set number of times that your PSA has to be tested in order to determine the rate of rise, although most researchers would agree that more frequent tests over longer periods of time will likely give a better sense of how your tumor is growing.

A rising PSA after surgery, radiation, or hormone treatment likely means that elements of the cancer remain in your system and need to be watched carefully, at a minimum, or subjected to further treatment. Ideally, the cancer would have been eradicated by the initial treatment(s), but that is not always the case.

In the event of a postsurgery detectable PSA, your oncologist will likely take one of several actions, which might include watchful waiting or a routine of ADT. The latter is usually administered by injection—plus oral tablets—and likely will be spread over a period of months, during which your blood will be tested regularly to measure the PSA and testosterone levels.

"Post-surgical PSA testing sometimes uses the ultrasensitive assay that in some labs measures down to 0.01," says Dana-Farber's Dr. Anthony V. D'Amico. At four to six weeks after surgery, a PSA baseline can be set. If at that time your doctor sees a rising PSA trend that exceeds 0.10, a doctor-patient discussion of other medical treatment is warranted.

More details of further potential treatments are presented in section 3, "What Are My Treatment Options?"

IN OUR OPINION. . .

Our opinions about prostate cancer and testing for it are succinctly stated: "Better safe than sorry"; caution is the byword. Thus, if your doctor says you should have an exam, have one. This is no time to second guess the coach.

The first step is PSA screening, and our position on this screening procedure aligns with the thinking of the American Urological Association, which is that the relative benefit of about a 20 percent reduction in disease-specific deaths could be very meaningful at the population level, explained next. The potential benefits of screening could extend beyond survival as a primary outcome and will depend on the relevant time horizon for each individual.

You should understand the difference between the "population level" and the test sample level. The population level means all 157 million males in the United States versus the small size of a test population, which could be a few hundred or a few thousand. In either case, one life in a thousand men is meaningful to us. The AUA also notes that: "The Panel concluded that PSA-based screening should not be performed in the absence of shared decision-making. *Thus, we recommend against organized screening in settings where shared decision-making is not part of routine practice (e.g., health fairs, health system promotions.)"*

We believe that testing for prostate cancer is critically important among men age fifty and older (or earlier if they are African American or have a family history of the disease). The test results then should be evaluated by your physician, who may refer you to an oncologist to differentiate true from false positives.

One false step could mean:

- *A seriously reduced quality of life for an otherwise healthy man*
- *An early death resulting from metastasized cancer, rather than an extended life*

Neither is desirable; so, be careful!

Section 2

CONTROVERSY AND DISAGREEMENT

9

The Controversy Continues:
To Test or Not to Test

For perspective, this chapter is divided into three sections that deal with PSA testing, a subject which is a very controversial among prostate cancer professionals worldwide. The sections that follow discuss the three major opinions or perspectives on cancer testing:

- *Major cancer organizations*
- *Major prostate cancer studies*
- *Divergent and nuanced policies on PSA screening*

Each section presents the arguments and statistics for both sides of the controversy—to test or not to test—that exist among professionals and institutions. The authors' own opinions are expressed at the end of each section in the "In Our Opinion. . ." summary. If you want to learn about what each study entails and their conclusions, read on. Otherwise, skip section 2 and move on to section 3.

MAJOR CANCER ORGANIZATIONS' OPINIONS ON TESTING

The American Cancer Society states that prostate cancer is the second leading cause of death in American men. African American men and men with family histories of prostate cancer have a higher chance of developing the disease.[1] Prostate cancer differs from some other cancers in that it tends to grow slowly. In 2020, 194,930 American men were diagnosed with prostate cancer, and over 33,3300 of them died from the disease, estimated the American Cancer Society.[2]

Despite decades of research and issuance of countless expert medical opinions about prostate cancer, a medical consensus on both testing and administering multiple levels of treatment for it has not yet emerged. There is no one correct course of action to detect and treat the disease, and perceptions of the value of testing for prostate cancer have been uneven.

For certain, however, the American Urological Association has taken a firm position: "The potential benefits of screening could extend beyond survival as a primary outcome and will depend on the relevant time horizon for an individual."[3] This means that the older a person is, the lower the potential positive impact that screening and treatment can have. Thus, men sixty-five and older may die of other causes before their prostate cancer can kill them.

As we have noted earlier, the professional journal *UpToDate states that prostate-specific antigen (PSA) testing was initially used to detect cancer recurrence or its progression following treatment, but now testing is employed as a means of screening for the presence of prostate cancer, which has led to an increase in the number of cases. UpToDate* also noted that increase in newly diagnosed cancers also led to an increase in radical prostatectomy and radiation therapy, aggressive treatments intended to cure these early-stage cancers. The *American Journal of Managed Care* reported that, "After the introduction of prostate-specific antigen (PSA) testing, the United States saw a dramatic increase in prostate cancer incidence between 1988 and 1992. Rates have decreased since then, with an accelerated decrease in more recent years."

Researchers have associated that decline in incidence with decreased PSA screening with the 2012 United States Preventive Services Task Force (USPSTF) recommendation against routine PSA screening. That organization is the dominant federal entity with an opinion on the efficacy of prostate cancer testing, and the 2017 Harvard *Annual Report on Prostate Cancer* called it "an influential volunteer panel of medical experts."[4] Its position on PSA screening, however, has wavered over time.[5]

"The USPSTF (in 2012) *discouraged PSA screening* for men of all ages, regardless of family history or race.[6] The recommendation was based on grade D evidence suggesting that the harms of testing outweigh the benefits," *Renal & Urology News* reported.[7] The USPSTF wrote that it "recommends against" PSA testing service because there is a

moderate or high certainty that the service [testing] has no net benefit or that the harms outweigh the benefits: Until we have better tests and better treatment options, based on a comprehensive review of the science, the USPSTF recommends that men not get the PSA test to screen for prostate cancer. [But] whether or not to be screened is a decision each man should make once he understands the facts and based on his own values and preferences.

The USPSTF added something of a disclaimer to its recommendation, however, just in case you chose to be tested in contravention to their recommendation: "You should know what the science says about PSA screening: There is a small potential benefit and there are significant potential harms," said NBC News quoting the USPSTF study.[8]

On the other hand, the American Urological Association's (AUA) opinion is much shorter, to the point, and differs significantly with the USPSTF. It states, "The benefits of PSA screening merit careful consideration" and says that "several studies have also revealed a significant reduction in prostate cancer specific mortality rates attributable to PSA-based screening for prostate cancer." And contrary to the opinion of the USPSTF, the AUA further notes, "One cannot ignore the benefits of earlier detection through screening in decreasing the risk of metastatic disease."[9]

In light of that, the following 2018 statement by the AUA ("Early Detection of Prostate Cancer") is extremely important:

The incidence of metastatic disease at presentation has declined by approximately three-fourths in the US since the advent of PSA screening. Further, in data from the [European study discussed below], the cumulative risk of metastatic disease at 9 to 11 years of follow-up was 31% to 33% lower in the screened arm compared to the control arm.[10] The [Swedish] arm of the trial demonstrated a 56% reduction in risk of metastatic disease.[11] Most of this reduction in metastatic disease was seen in cancers detected at the time of diagnosis in the screened arm and not following diagnosis.

The AUA summarized its position regarding prostate cancer screening, stating that the relative benefit could be very meaningful at the population level.[12] The "relative benefits" they write of are a 20 percent reduction in disease-specific deaths at the "population level," which of course is much larger than the study universe. "The potential benefits of screening could extend beyond survival as a primary outcome," it stated, which means that the older a person is when he is diagnosed, the less time will be available for problems to develop.[13]

In support of the advantage of early diagnosis of prostate cancer—thus before metastases—the American Cancer Society cites National Cancer Institute conclusions relative to local-, regional-, and distant-stage cancers.[14]

- "Local stage means that there is no sign that the cancer has spread outside of the prostate. . . . About 4 out of 5 prostate cancers are found in this early stage. The relative 5-year survival rate for local stage prostate cancer is nearly 100%.
- "Regional stage means the cancer has spread from the prostate to nearby areas. . . . The relative 5-year survival rate for regional stage prostate cancer is nearly 100%.
- "Distant stage includes . . . cancers that have spread to distant lymph nodes, bones, or other organs. The relative five-year survival rate for distant stage prostate cancer is about 29%."

IN OUR OPINION. . .

We believe that broad-brush approach of the USPSTF and its generalized expansion of PSA testing have been interpreted to favor limited testing—which we believe is inappropriate. We maintain that such a limited-testing approach that restricts PSA testing:

1. *Undervalues a doctor's ability to exercise caution and wise use of his educated judgment.*
2. *Underestimates a patient's desires to maintain quality of life outcomes, which can be significant and include impotence and both forms of incontinence, plus numerous other negative reactions.*

Thus, we believe that when a doctor exercises cautious judgment, and a patient expresses an understanding of the importance of quality of life, then the patient's own decision-making abilities will ensure his optimum outcome—especially when aided by a personal decision assistant (such assistants are discussed later in this book).

Supporting our conclusion is the AUA statement that, "Several studies have also revealed a significant reduction in prostate cancer specific mortality rates attributable to PSA-based screening for prostate cancer." The association further notes, "One cannot ignore the benefits of earlier detection through screening in decreasing the risk of metastatic disease."[15] *This means that screening has a measurable positive result in catching prostate cancer when it is localized in the prostate and has not spread to other parts of the body. As noted earlier, once the cancer has metastasized, the chances of death from prostate cancer are virtually 100 percent, an outcome no one wants.*

MAJOR PROSTATE CANCER STUDY FINDINGS

Globally, three prostate cancer studies have emerged as important influences in assessing the apparent efficacy of various efforts at screening and treating the disease. These are the European Randomized Study for Prostate Cancer (ERSPC); the Göteborg [Sweden] Randomized Population-based Prostate Cancer Screening; and in the United States, the Prostate, Lung, Colorectal and Ovarian Cancer Screening Trial (PLCO). For a variety of reasons, the ERSPC is considered the work that provides benchmark results.

The three studies, and other opinions as well, point to a fear that overscreening for prostate cancer can lead to overtreating for it, which can have significant and potentially negative physiological and psychological outcomes. And those ills may be lifelong. At the same time, experts express a concern with undertesting, which can allow an otherwise localized prostate cancer to spread to other parts of the body, thus, to metastasize. This assuredly causes lifelong, and often fatal, consequences.

The American Urological Association concludes: "One cannot ignore the benefits of earlier detection through screening in decreasing the risk of metastatic disease."[16]

The European Randomized Study of Screening for Prostate Cancer

The ERSPC began screening European men ages fifty to seventy-four; however, by the end of the thirteen-year analysis, the 162,243 men in the study were between the ages of fifty-five and sixty-nine.

A significant outcome of screening was that death was 21 percent lower in that group. The absolute rates of prostate cancer mortality were 0.43 versus 0.54 per one thousand person-years. While the ~20 percent difference appears to be relatively small, when expanded to a population level, it becomes significant. It is particularly significant if you are among those men who comprise that 20 percent; it means life or death.

The professional medical journal *UpToDate* commented on the study's results and went beyond the 20 percent improvement in mortality, suggesting the following:

Although the absolute mortality benefit for screening was low, several factors could have biased the results. . . . Adjusting for contamination and non-adherence with screening [guidelines], investigators estimated that prostate cancer screening could reduce prostate cancer mortality by as much as 31%.

The publication had a warning, however: "Furthermore, while the prostate cancer survival benefit from screening was not initially realized until nine years of follow-up, the burdens of screening and treatment, including harms from over-diagnosis and over-treatment, occur immediately and potentially have lifelong consequences."[17] In short, the European study provided evidence that screening for prostate cancer can provide significant positive outcomes in terms of both detection and extended lifespan, especially at a population level.

Corroborating *UpToDate*'s comments on the ERSPC study results, the *Asian Journal of Urology* summarized them as such: "After 13 years of follow-up, the trial showed that PC [prostate cancer] mortality was reduced by 21% in favor of the screening arm."[18]

The American Urological Association spoke out with statistics on this subject as well, saying, "Once diagnosed with prostate cancer, a man is faced with the risk of overtreatment of indolent [slowly developing, non-threatening] disease due to the assumption that diagnosis with a malignancy must necessarily result in treatment of this malignancy." It also noted, however, that "Estimates of over-diagnosis vary widely," from less than 5 percent to more than 75 percent. The AUA added, however, that while its own estimate of actual overtreatment is "closer to that seen with breast and colon cancer screening, the risk of overtreatment remains a valid concern due to the impact of treatment on Quality of Life."[19]

The British Association of Urological Surgeons takes a more skeptical view: "The ERSPC study demonstrates a 20% survival benefit surprisingly early in follow-up. However, this is at the cost of considerable over-treatment and, hence, significant side-effects in a group of men, most of who would not die from prostate cancer."

The AUA acknowledges the concern of screening critics, writing: "Quality of Life may be impaired as a result [of unnecessary testing] due to lasting impairment in urinary, bowel and sexual function. Thus, personal preferences should play a large role in both a decision to screen and in prostate cancer management if diagnosed."

One form or another of the term "personal preference" crops up in almost every report with respect to prostate cancer screening outcomes. The prevalence of this cautionary phrase underscores the belief that the male patient population is not fully, or even adequately, informed about their detection and treatment options and the implications of their choices. Thus, we believe that the assistance and insight of an informed personal decision assistant is desirable, and this option is discussed in section 4 of this book.

The Göteborg Randomized Population-Based Prostate Cancer Screening

In the Göteborg trial, many of the men in the test sample were also ERSPC participants. The Swedish study classified fifty- to sixty-four-year-old men into two groups: an "organized screening" group and an "opportunistic testing" group. Population registries were used to select the participants, who were randomly allocated to one of the two groups.

Data from the Göteborg study "corroborate previous findings that systematic PSA screening reduces prostate cancer mortality and suggest that systematic screening may reduce socio-demographic inequality in mortality."[20] The fourteen-year study included 19,904 men and, according to the *Asian Journal of Urology*, concluded that:

- "Systematic PSA screening demonstrated greater benefit in PC mortality for men who started screening at age 55–59 years.

- "The Goteborg Randomized Prostate Cancer Screening Trial . . . showed that PCA mortality decreased by 44% in the screening group as compared to the control group."[21]

Consistent with the opinions of other observers, the British Association of Urological Surgeons said, "The Göteborg group, published in *Lancet Oncology*, had longer follow-up, an earlier onset for screening and a slightly lower PSA threshold for biopsy. This study showed clearly that PSA testing saves lives from prostate cancer."[22, 23] The number needed to screen and treat were lower. Importantly, about a third of the men with low-risk prostate cancer stayed on monitoring programs, demonstrating that early diagnosis does not necessarily translate into "overtreatment."

The United States Prostate, Lung, Colorectal, and Ovarian Cancer Screening Study

The PLCO study, as it's called, was conducted among 76,693 men between the ages of fifty-five and seventy-four. They were randomly assigned to annual screenings with PSA and digital rectal exams (DRE) or to routine care that did not include either of those. Unfortunately, a number of factors biased the PLCO trial toward a null result.

Despite the reported fact that cancer detection in the screening group was significantly higher than in the control group (2,820 versus 2,322), "investigators found no evidence that screening could be beneficial in any subgroups defined by co-morbidity, age, or pre-trial PSA testing," according to *UpToDate*.[24] Indeed, after seven years of follow-up, *there was no reduction in the primary outcome of prostate cancer mortality* of fifty versus forty-four deaths in the screening and control groups, respectively.

Why is this so? Why were the US results so different from those in Europe? *UpToDate* speculates that negative [US] results are most likely attributable to the "very high rate of PSA testing" in the United States, which has been estimated as high as 80 percent, and to the high proportion of subjects with recent PSA testing at baseline.

Consistent with the opinions of other observers, the British Association of Urological Surgeons said, "The PLCO trial failed to show a benefit for additional screening in an already heavily-screened population.

It is likely that this so-called "contamination" of the control arm markedly reduced the power of the study, hence "few conclusions can be drawn."

Conclusions from These Studies

The *American Urology Association Journal* examined these studies and reported the following:

> Prostate cancer specific mortality was the primary endpoint for both the ERSPC and the PLCO trials. However, one cannot ignore the benefits of earlier detection through screening in decreasing the risk of metastatic disease.[25] The incidence of metastatic disease at presentation has declined by approximately three-fourths [75%] in the US since the advent of PSA screening. Further, in data from the ERSPC, the cumulative risk of metastatic disease at 9 to 11 years of follow-up was 31% to 33% lower in the screened arm compared to the control arm.[26, 27] The Goteborg arm of the trial demonstrated a 56% reduction in risk of metastatic disease. Most of this reduction in metastatic disease was seen in cancers detected at the time of diagnosis in the screened arm and not following diagnosis.[28]

UpToDate also reported that "Apart from issues of cost and acceptability, in order for prostate cancer screening to be valuable, it must reduce disease-specific morbidity and/or mortality."[29]

IN OUR OPINION. . .

Despite vacillating recommendations of the USPSTF, we believe that regular, cautious prostate screening is beneficial in the detection of early-stage prostate cancer and the reduction of metastasized prostate cancer.

We come to this conclusion based on the findings of the European Randomized Study for Prostate Cancer, ERSPC; the Göteborg [Sweden] Randomized Population-Based Prostate Cancer Screening; and (to a lesser degree) the Prostate, Lung, Colorectal and Ovarian Cancer Screening Trial, PLCO.

While there exists a reasonable fear that overscreening for prostate cancer can lead to overtreatment, experts are also concerned with undertesting, which can allow a localized prostate cancer to metasta-size to other parts of the body, which is incurable and often fatal.

Furthermore, the American Urological Association concludes that, "One cannot ignore the benefits of earlier detection through screening in decreasing the risk of metastatic disease."[30]

We believe that risks exist in both action and inaction. With careful and regular examination (testing/screening) followed by enlightened medical judgment and cautious action, however, the benefits of testing for prostate cancer significantly outweigh the outcomes a man may experience in the absence of such efforts.

DIVERGENT AND NUANCED POLICIES ON PSA SCREENING

Corporate and governmental perspectives and policies can have a significant impact on ways a disease is approached—by both men at risk and their doctors. While quality of life should always be an issue, it is not uncommon for a physician to be clinically focused on a nar-row realm, treating one specific problem, then moving on to the next specific problem. This singular focus obviates a broader, more holis-tic approach, which considers the entire person, not merely a single condition.

Since testing (screening) and treating for prostate cancer are very personal issues, governmental and institutional policies that guide or limit access to medical services can also become very personal issues. Therefore, in this section, we will look at variations in governmental and institutional policies and the implications of these policies on your pros-tate cancer treatment outcomes—and potential harms for you and other American men.

Because there are numerous opinions about prostate cancer and its detection and treatment, we provide an overview of several of those on the following pages. However, this level of detail may not appeal to all readers, therefore you may want to skip to the "In Our Opinion. . ." section.

Before we review the numerous opinions on screening, the American Urological Association (see its 2018 position on "Early Detection of Prostate Cancer") creates an important context in which to consider all screening activities:

The Panel [in 2012] concluded that PSA-based screening should not be performed in the absence of shared-decision making. Thus, we recommend against organized screening in settings where shared-decision making is not part of routine practice (e.g., health fairs, health system promotions, community organizations).

The detection of possible or actual prostate cancer is very serious and can result in meaningful and negative physiological and psychological impacts. Therefore, dealing with it should not be a casual experience.

The US Government's USPSTF Position

The US Preventive Services Task Force's recommendation in favor of screening in 2008 launched a surge in PSA testing, but only four years later, in May 2012, it changed its position and opposed PSA screening, stating: "The USPSTF concludes that there is moderate certainty that the benefits of PSA-based screening for prostate cancer do not outweigh the harms."[31]

By the spring of 2017, however, the USPSTF once again changed its advice, stating:

> The USPSTF recommends that clinicians inform men ages 55 to 69 years about the potential benefits and harms of prostate-specific antigen (PSA)–based screening for prostate cancer. The decision about whether to be screened for prostate cancer should be an individual one. . . . The USPSTF recommends individualized decision-making about screening for prostate cancer after discussion with a clinician, so that each man has an opportunity to understand the potential benefits and harms of screening and to incorporate his values and preferences into his decision.[32]

The USPSTF assigned a grade of C to prostate cancer testing, revising its earlier grade of D. The task force maintained its D grade for testing of men seventy years of age and older.

Six Opinions in the United States Medical Community

- American Academy of Family Physicians "recommends against prostate-specific antigen testing to screen for prostate cancer because the harms outweigh the benefits in most men."[33]

- American Cancer Society recommends that men "make an informed decision (about screening) with their healthcare provider." The screening decision thresholds are:
  - Age forty if a man is in the high-risk group, thus "a first-degree family member had prostate cancer."
  - Age forty-five with a moderate risk, thus black men or those with first-degree kin having had prostate cancer.
  - Age fifty, thus men expected to live ten or more years.
- American College of Physicians concludes: "In men 55 to 74 years of age, annual screening with prostate-specific antigen testing and digital rectal examination did not reduce mortality from prostate cancer."[34]
- American College of Preventive Medicine recommends that clinicians discuss the potential benefits and harms of PSA screening with men age fifty or older, consider their patients' preferences, and individualize screening decisions.
- American Urological Association sidles up to the USPSTF and covers all its bases with a three-point "Guideline Statement":
  - One, the panel "recommends against PSA screening in men under the age of 40."
  - Two, it "does not recommend routine screening in men between ages 40 to 54" (except for men with a family history of prostate cancer or who are African American).
  - Three, for men fifty-five to sixty-nine, the AUA panel of experts "strongly recommends shared decision-making."[35]
- Centers for Disease Control and Prevention, a US government agency, takes a noncommittal position and ultimately throws the issue back to the attending physician: "A PSA test can find prostate cancer earlier than no screening at all. However, the PSA test may have false positive or false negative results. . . . Talk to your doctor about the right decision for you."[36]

The Canadian Position

The Canadian Task Force on Preventive Health Care "recommends against screening for prostate cancer with the PSA test. It found that the potentially small benefit from PSA screening is outweighed by the potentially significant harms of the screening and associated follow-up treatment.[37]

The British Position

The British Association of Urological Surgeons (BAUS) states: "Overall, the evidence for screening is not yet sufficient to recommend it as a national program. However, that decision is much more finely balanced than the consultation [UK National Screening Committee] would suggest. In addition, BAUS remains extremely concerned by data from the prostate charities, which show that a significant number of men requesting PSA testing are refused the test by their GP (personal physician)."

The UK's National Health Service says, "*There is no national screening programme* for prostate cancer because we don't have a reliable enough test to use. Current tests have risks."[38, 39]

A Sampling of American Insurance Companies

In the United States, insurance companies are *regulated on a state-by-state* basis, and as stated by Blue Cross Blue Shield of Rhode Island: "Benefits may vary between groups/contracts." Because of the likelihood for disparity among insurers and individual states, the following are *merely representative* statements on PCA screening.

- Aetna Insurance: "Aetna considers prostate-specific antigen (PSA) screening a medically necessary preventive service for men aged 40 years and older. . . . When used for routine screening, annual PSA screening is considered medically necessary. . . . Aetna considers diagnostic PSA testing medically necessary for men of all ages with signs or symptoms of prostate cancer, and for follow-up of men with prostate cancer." [40]
- Blue Cross Blue Shield of Illinois addresses the question without taking a stand: "While the USPSTF recommends against PSA-based screening for prostate cancer, the American Cancer Society (ACS) and the American Urological Association (AUA) recommend an informed decision-making process for men age 50 and older (ACS) for men age 55–69 (AUA) who have at least a ten-year life expectancy. Among the potential considerations for informed

decision-making are the risks, benefits and uncertainties of screening, as well as individual values and preferences. ACS states that prostate cancer screening should not occur without an informed decision-making process."

- CIGNA of Texas states that most Cigna-insured health benefit plans include coverage for each covered male for an annual medically recognized diagnostic examination for the detection of prostate cancer. Those benefits include:
  - A physical examination for the detection of prostate cancer
  - A PSA test for each covered male who is "at least 50 years of age; or at least 40 years of age with a family history of prostate cancer or other prostate cancer risk factor."[41]

Since annual PSA screening is controversial even among healthcare professionals, insurance companies, national healthcare agencies, and practitioners themselves, the alternative is simply monitoring a man's condition, otherwise known as watchful waiting. However, such monitoring may prove to be the most dangerous course, as pointed out by one of the nation's leading radiation oncologists specializing in prostate cancer treatment, Dr. Anthony V. D'Amico, of Boston's Dana-Farber Cancer Institute:

"I think it much better to have a test that finds everything and let the doctors figure out what needs to be treated and what doesn't need to be treated, rather than have a test that either finds it when it is too late or only finds a portion of those [individuals] that need to be cured."[42]

IN OUR OPINION. . .

We believe that the opinions of noted medical experts and of respected medical organizations show that the positive results derived from early, regular, and cautious testing for prostate cancer outweighs the often-serious outcomes—including metastasizes—that may accrue from withholding such testing.

Our conclusion is based on opinions offered by:

- *European Randomized Study for Prostate Cancer*

- *Göteborg, Sweden, Randomized Population-based Prostate Cancer Screening*
- *The American Urological Association, which says: "One cannot ignore the benefits of earlier detection through screening in decreasing the risk of metastatic disease."*[43]
- *The Prostate, Lung, Colorectal and Ovarian Cancer Screening Trial in the United States.*

We find the position taken by Aetna in 2018 to be correct: "Aetna considers prostate-specific antigen (PSA) screening a medically necessary preventive service for men aged 40 years and older. . . . When used for routine screening, annual PSA screening is considered medically necessary. . . . Aetna considers diagnostic PSA testing medically necessary for men of all ages with signs or symptoms of prostate cancer, and for follow-up of men with prostate cancer."[44]

Section 3

WHAT ARE MY TREATMENT OPTIONS?

10

Early-Stage Treatment Options
and Their Implications

What begins with a simple blood test and the subsequent PSA assessment can end in a complex array of tests, terminologies, and behaviors—most, if not all, of which will be new and strange to the male patient and his family.

While many of these treatments may seem benign at the outset, it is unlikely that they will end that way. Many patients involved in treatments for prostate cancer will suffer meaningful changes in their daily lives.

The following are the possible treatments you will encounter at the direction of your oncology team—specialists in surgery, hormone or chemical administration, and radiology, among others. While not all patients will have difficulty enduring the treatments, many will suffer incontinence or impotence, some for a few months, or years, or forever following treatment.

The traditional doctor-patient relationship is clinical; it is a service-provider/customer relationship, where the doctor is laser-focused on eliminating or mitigating a patient's problem.

Indeed, doctor specialists tends to be highly focused on their area of unique expertise, sometimes irrespective of what might be the ideal treatment for a patient's condition based on a 1998 survey of over one thousand radiation oncologists and urologists in the United States. According to Anthony Zeeman, author of *Counseling the Patient with Prostate Cancer,* that survey revealed "depressing results" that showed the "truly 'partisan' nature" of cancer specialists: for example, 93 percent of surgeons recommended surgery as primary therapy for early-stage prostate cancer, and 72 percent of radiation oncologists recommended radiation.[1] Such narrowly-focused approaches—surgeons favoring surgery and radiologists favoring radiology—should change dramatically, as prostate cancer requires a relationship between multiple medical disciplines, but that seems not to be the case.

EMPLOYING A MULTIDISCIPLINARY APPROACH

Since the implications of the doctor successfully accomplishing his "job" are far-reaching, we believe that a multidisciplinary approach to prostate cancer treatment has considerable benefit.

As a result of the National Cancer Act of 1971, the National Institutes of Health recognizes seventy-one NCI-Designated Cancer Centers in thirty-six states and the District of Columbia. All of them "meet rigorous standards for trans-disciplinary, state-of-the-art research focused on developing new and better approaches to preventing, diagnosing and treating cancer."[2] (A list of NCI-Designated Cancer Centers and Cooperative Groups appears in the Resources section.)

These centers "develop and translate scientific knowledge from promising laboratory discoveries into new treatments for cancer patients," including those with prostate cancer. The advantages of the multidisciplinary, or team approach to prostate cancer treatment should be obvious: multiple cancer clinicians and specialists gather to assess and recommend a course of treatment. Among those assembled are experts in radiation oncology, urologic surgery, medical oncology, radiology, pathology, psychological, and physiological, among others.

There are two methods of delivering this approach: internal and external. With the internal method, experts often review individually or in subgroups the patients' records and test results, then collectively commence a course of treatment. In the external method, clinicians meet in a group to review the same data that was reviewed by the internal, on-site group to determine the course of treatment. This latter approach is used by the Prostate Cancer Multidisciplinary Clinic at Johns Hopkins, and by Humanitis, in Milan, Italy, which is considered a leader in European cancer care. Other cancer centers in the United States have similar programs.

The Johns Hopkins approach as indicative of American care begins with patient consultation that includes the following:[3]

- Review with the patient of all treatments that are available to him at the facility.
- Comprehensive case assessments, including appropriate records and studies.
- Collective expert consultations and evaluations, and potential treatment options.
- Written reports of the experts' conclusions provided to your referring physician.
- Educational materials provided to the patient and his family.

The Humanitis approach is quite similar. To prepare a man and his spouse or partner for the certain changes that will come with his treatment—surgery, radiation, hormone therapy, or something else—the Italian facility has initiated pre- and post-treatment regimes designed to help ensure patients understanding of what is about to happen, or has just happened, to them. Humanitis has been granted "Research Hospital" status by the Italian Ministry of Health, which says that its facility is "considered one of the most technologically advanced hospitals in Europe."[4]

As with NIH-designated hospitals, the Humanitis goal is to provide a man and his family with "a place where any doubts they may have can be resolved." Accordingly,

A month before undergoing the procedure, patients are invited to an informational meeting with surgeons, nurses and two other individuals who will [continue to] play a role after the surgery. The individuals include a rehabilitator for the pelvic floor and an andrologist for male sexual function. The patient must be aware of two issues that might arise after the surgery. These include urinary incontinence and decreased sexual function."

This group approach, the hospital says, "helps break down the barriers that characterize the relationship between doctor and patient. The aim of the counseling is to provide the patient with quality care even before he enters the hospital, resolve any doubts he may have, and make him feel closer to the medical team in charge of his case."

Patients and their partners attend the first counseling session, which is attended by:

- Urologists, who show the characteristics and peculiarities associated with robot-assisted prostatectomy.
- Nurses, who explain practical aspects of the operation ("from the insertion of the catheter, the choice of pajamas, and preoperative hair removal").
- A physical therapist, who explains rehabilitation following the operation.
- Another physician, who presents the andrological point of view, defined as "a branch of medicine concerned with the anatomy, functions, and disorders, such as infertility or impotence of the male reproductive system."
- Sometimes a patient who had already undergone a prostatectomy to speak about his experience.

Humanitis is considered one of the most technologically advanced hospitals in Europe.[5] It is accredited by the National Health Service of Italy, and combines specialized centers for the treatment of cancers, cardiovascular diseases, and neurological and orthopedic disorders, as well as an Ophthalmology Centre and a Fertility Center.

What Humanitis has initiated is a form of multidisciplinary care, which appears to be increasingly the standard for cancer care in the United States. It has long been the practice of medical professionals to meet among themselves to evaluate a prostate cancer patient's care and decide who among them should lead at each stage of treatment. This could be considered a form of "interdisciplinary care" practiced efficiently in the background. This, however, is quite different than the up-front, fully transparent meetings that Humanitis practices, where such a multidisciplinary group meets with the prostate cancer patient before the beginning of treatment and continues such meetings during and after treatment.

The Dartmouth-Norris Cotton Cancer Center at the Dartmouth-Hitchcock Medical Center, on the other hand, expresses the objective and practice of "interdisciplinary care" succinctly:

> In an interdisciplinary clinic, experts in diagnosing and treating specific types of cancers come together to provide personalized, complete cancer care, all through one point of contact, at one location. Whenever possible, individual visits with several providers may be coordinated on a single day, which eliminates long delays between appointments.

Dartmouth-Hitchcock's Norris Cotton Cancer Center states that its "ultimate goal" in practicing an interdisciplinary approach is:

- "See the right medical staff in the right order.
- Get the necessary tests with timely and accurate results.
- Understand the diagnosis and the best treatment options.
- Have complete support throughout the process."

"The use of multidisciplinary strategies among in-hospital teams limits adverse events, improves outcomes, and adds to patient and employee satisfaction," according to the National Institutes of Health.[6] "Delivering the best medical/surgical care is a 'team sport'" that achieves the Dartmouth center's goals and also maximizes patient safety and satisfaction, decreases the length of a patient's stay in the hospital, and increases the quality of treatment outcomes. Further benefits, especially to the hospital or clinic, include optimizing worker performance, reducing hospital costs and complications, and increasing job satisfaction.

The NIH says that this multifaceted approach to delivering healthcare:

Should remind hospital administrators of the critical need to keep mul-tidisciplinary teams together, so that they can continue to operate their "well-oiled machines" enhancing the quality/safety of patient care, while enabling 'staff' to optimize their performance and enhance their job satisfaction.

You might say, when we all work together, we all work better together. And the patient benefits from that coordinated effort. "Treatments vary according to the type of prostate cancer, its stage and the risk of the cancer spreading" according to Dr. Sean Cavanaugh, Chief of Radiation Oncology and Medical Director of the Prostate Center at the Cancer Treatment Centers of America in Atlanta.[7] "I think a man who's edu-cated about what's going on in his body is more likely to make a healthy decision for him and his family," he says.

Indeed, the University of California at San Francisco offers the same prudent advice:

Some prostate cancers grow quickly and spread—or metastasize—to other parts of the body. If unchecked, these cancers can be fatal. Most prostate cancers, however, are slow growing and in many cases, immediate treatment isn't necessary. Many men take several months to decide what to do. The decision can be complicated. You should consider the pros and cons of the various treatments, get second opinions and decide what is best for you, all of which may take time.[8]

Thoughtful review and consideration of the benefits and risks of each treatment will help a patient and his partner make an informed decision. Research shows that the better informed a patient is before and during his decision-making process, the more likely he is to accept and be satisfied with the outcomes.

Your decision of which treatment(s) to choose will depend on a variety of factors, and the University of California San Francisco (UCSF) recommends considering two overriding factors:

First, evaluate yourself and the progression of your cancer, which may include:

• The cancer's stage and grade
• Your age and life expectancy
• Your overall health and other medical needs
• The cost of the treatment, and to what degree will insurance cover it
• Your attitude about a cure or "living with cancer"
• Your own needs, interpersonal relationships, and values

Second, whether the cancer is confined to the prostate or has spread to other parts of your body—metastasized—will have considerable impact on your decisions about treatment. The UCSF warns, however, that "in many cases, it is difficult to know definitively whether or not the cancer is confined to the prostate. This uncertainty may arise in cases when the cancer is at a higher state (T2b or above), and/or has a Gleason score of 7 or more, and/or has a pretreatment PSA above 10" (see the Gleason score discussion earlier in this book).[9]

In any case, *patient counseling* by trained practitioners is valuable and is increasingly available in many parts of the United States, and we believe that counseling should be considered by all men facing the significant decisions related to living with prostate cancer as well as living with the results of treatment.

TREATMENT OPTIONS

The following is a list of treatment options, then a brief discussion of each.

1. Surgery
   a. Radical prostatectomy
   b. Laparoscopic Prostatectomy
2. Radiation therapy
   a. External beam radiation
   b. Brachytherapy
3. Cryosurgery
4. Hormone therapy
5. Intermittent hormone therapy
6. Chemotherapy
7. Active surveillance
8. Clinical trials
9. Alternative therapies

Surgery

Radical Prostatectomy

Surgery has long been regarded as the "gold standard" in prostate cancer treatment, according to the University of California in San Francisco. It is used most often when your doctor believes your prostate cancer has not spread beyond the gland itself. The procedure removes the prostate gland and surrounding tissue. The surgery is done under general anesthesia, generally takes two to four hours, and requires a hospital stay of two to three days.

While radical prostatectomy has been performed successfully for many years, there is still no guarantee that the cancer will not return. One value of a prostatectomy is that the primary tumor is removed and can be fully examined by the pathologist, which provides a more complete assessment of the tumor than a mere sample from a needle biopsy.

A radical prostatectomy can be either nerve-sparing or nonnerve-sparing. After a nerve-sparing procedure, the impotence rate drops to between 25 to 30 percent for men under age sixty. After a non-nerve-sparing radical prostatectomy, about 90 percent of men become impotent. Medications and treatments such as Viagra, penile injection procedures, and counseling have helped men deal with erectile dysfunction.

While urinary incontinence is also a problematic side effect, bladder control may return within several weeks or a few months. From 1 percent to 5 percent of patients have permanent stress incontinence during coughing, laughing, sneezing, or exercising.

"Kegel exercises" may improve or restore bladder control. While the effectiveness of Kegel exercises is debated among those in the medical community (and patients), we discuss the subject in more detail beginning in the Urinary Incontinence chapter later in this book.

Potential short- and long-term side effects of a radical prostatectomy are the following:

- Impotence
- Urinary incontinence
- Fecal incontinence
- Pain during orgasm
- Shortening of the penis

Laparoscopic Prostatectomy

While the laparoscopic surgery procedure has been around for a long time, it wasn't until 2016 that the Cleveland Clinic began its use in prostate procedures. The clinic claims to have "the most experience of any healthcare center in the United States related to laparoscopic prostatectomy."[10]

Traditional prostate cancer surgery for tumor removal requires about an eight-inch incision; the minimally invasive laparoscopic version, on the other hand, requires four or five small incisions—each about half an inch or less—for surgical entrustments to enter your body. It's also known as keyhole, porthole, or minimally invasive surgery.[11] The laparoscopic method "offers surgeons an unparalleled visualization of the pelvic area, thus permitting precise removal of the prostate" and less loss of a patient's blood, according to the Cleveland Clinic.

The advantages of Laparoscopy are several, writes *Web*MD, and include the following.[12]

1. Patients have shortened hospital stays, down to one to two days depending on how quickly you recover from the surgery. *Web*MD says that about half of the men who undergo this form of treatment are discharged one day after surgery.
2. Patients have reduced bleeding.
3. Patients require fewer, and perhaps no, painkillers.
4. The catheter is often removed a week or two after surgery.
5. About 90 percent of patients return to full activity within two or three weeks.

Potential short- and long-term side effects are the following:

1. Urinary and sometimes fecal incontinence
2. Occasional bladder spasms
3. Impotence, erectile dysfunction

Radiation Therapy

Radiation therapy sends high-energy rays, usually X-rays, to tumors to kill cancer cells. There are two main types: External Beam Radiation Therapy and Brachytherapy, or seed implantation.

External Beam Radiation

External beam radiation treatment, which last only a few minutes, is typically delivered at a medical facility for each of five weekdays over a period of seven to eight weeks. 3D conformal radiation therapy, an advanced form of external beam radiation, reduces the radiation received by nearby tissues while concentrating the radiation dose at the cancer site. It maps the prostate gland precisely so that radiation beams can attack it from up to six or seven different directions.

Another approach to this method is Intensity Modulated Radiation Therapy, IMRT, which can vary the intensity of the radiation beams, according to UCSF. It is an advanced type of radiation therapy used to treat both cancerous and noncancerous tumors. According to the Mayo Clinic, "IMRT uses advanced technology to manipulate photon and proton beams of radiation to conform to the shape of a tumor. . . . "IMRT uses multiple small photon or proton beams of varying intensities to precisely irradiate a tumor. The radiation intensity of each beam is controlled, and the beam shape changes throughout each treatment."[13]

This proton beam radiation therapy, using protons instead of the traditional X-rays, is "presently available at only a few centers in this country," according to the UCSF. "Studies have shown that proton beam therapy is effective in treating localized prostate cancer. However, the data is inconclusive as to whether proton therapy yields better outcomes than X-ray therapy."

Brachytherapy

Brachytherapy, also known as seed implantation, involves placing radioactive gold seeds into the prostate. This method allows a radiation oncologist to very precisely deliver the radiation treatment. It has two forms of treatment: a permanent seed implant (SI) and a temporary method called high-dose rate brachytherapy (HDR).

In the SI method, which is an outpatient procedure, radioactive pellets, or "seeds," about the size of a grain of rice, are implanted into the prostate. They will give off radiation for a few months.

In the HDR method, radioactive material is placed in the prostate for relatively short periods of time, then withdrawn. Two to three treatments are to be expected during a one- to two-day hospital stay.

External beam radiational and brachytherapy have the potential following short-term side effects:

- Fatigue
- Urinary leakage
- Increased urinary frequency
- Mild to moderate burning during urination
- Rectal bleeding and inflammation of the rectum
- Abdominal cramping
- Diarrhea
- About 40 to 60 percent of men who receive external beam radiation therapy develop some degree of impotence (the inability to achieve an erection a year or more after the treatment). The risk might be higher if they receive hormonal treatment.[14]

External beam radiation's potential long-term side effects include:

- Erectile dysfunction
- Fecal incontinence
- Urinary incontinence
- Rectal bleeding
- Secondary cancers in treated areas

Brachytherapy has the following potential short-term side effects:

- Pain
- Blood in urine
- Burning during urination
- Frequent urination
- Urinary retention

Brachytherapy has the following potential long-term side effects:

- Impotence
- Rectal bleeding.
- Narrowing of the urethra

Cryosurgery

Cryosurgery freezes prostate cancer cells to kill them. The University of California at San Francisco says that, "This method has shown good results in treating cancer confined to the prostate but is presently performed at a limited number of locations around the country."[15]

Cryosurgery is a minimally invasive approach to prostate cancer in which "surgeons insert needles into the prostate to freeze and destroy the prostate cancer cells. Argon and helium gases circulate through the needles, lowering the temperature to –40°C for several minutes. Surgeons can control the extent of freezing and evaluate the prostate and needle placement with real-time ultrasound imaging during the procedure," according to the New York-Presbyterian Hospital/Columbia University Medical Center's Department of Urology.[16]

Compared with such surgical procedures as radical prostatectomy, cryosurgery is "less invasive and causes fewer side effects. Also, cryosurgery is a recognized option for patients who fail after primary radio- or cryotherapy and have localized recurrence and has been shown to provide very good cancer control and functional outcomes" according to the Medical Center.

Since cryosurgery is usually performed as an outpatient procedure, patients go home the day of treatment, and recovery is rapid. "Cryosurgery entails a lower risk of side effects such as incontinence. And for some men cryosurgery results in minimal damage to the nerves involved in sexual function," thus reducing the chance of impotence, according to Columbia University Medical Center.

However, some medical professionals believe that to achieve maximum effectiveness from cryosurgery, the whole prostate must be frozen, which "has a negative impact on nerve bundles on the sides of the gland. Therefore, impotence almost always results from cryosurgery when the entire gland is treated. Urinary incontinence also may occur," according to UCSF, which also says, "Some physicians are performing 'focal' cryotherapy, where only the cancerous area of the prostate is treated, in patients where color Doppler imaging indicates the presence of very limited disease. There is the risk that microscopic amounts of cancer may be missed, and studies have shown mixed results with this approach. When appropriate, cryosurgery can be repeated if the cancer recurs."[17]

Hormone Therapy

Hormone therapy is a common treatment for prostate cancer, but the full understanding of what it entails and the broad extent of the outcomes produced by the process may not be fully understood by patients.

Since this is a complex and important aspect of prostate cancer treatment, let's start with a simple definition:

> Androgen is any of a group of hormones that primarily influence the growth and development of the male reproductive system. The predominant and most active androgen is testosterone, which is produced by the male testes, but is also made by the ovaries and the adrenal gland.[18]

In April 2019, the American Cancer Society wrote that hormone therapy might be used in the following situations:[19]

1. If the cancer has spread too far to be cured by surgery or radiation, or if you can't have these treatments for some other reason.

2. If the cancer remains or comes back after treatment with surgery or radiation therapy.
3. Along with radiation therapy as an initial treatment if you are at higher risk of the cancer coming back after treatment (based on a high Gleason score, high PSA level, and/or growth of the cancer outside the prostate).
4. Before radiation to try to shrink the cancer to make treatment more effective.

"Most prostate cancers are very responsive to hormone therapy when first diagnosed," according to the UCSF.[20] "Hormone therapy usually is recommended as the initial treatment for advanced prostate cancers, including prostate cancers that have metastasized. Hormone therapy does have significant side effects, and the decision to undergo it should not be made casually."

All men considering initiating a course of hormone therapy must remember that such action will have *significant implications*. But, unfortunately, hormone therapy "seems to be less well understood by patients even though their lives will be significantly altered," as the ACS notes in its "Hormone Therapy for Prostate Cancer." Because of the potential extensive side effects of ADT—including, but not limited to, impotence and urinary and fecal incontinence—the decision to select this option must be taken *very seriously* and with good counsel.

The objective of hormone therapy is to reduce levels of male hormones called androgens in the body, or to stop them from stimulating prostate cancer cells. Hormone therapy may also shrink the cancer or lower the risk of an early return of prostate cancer after treatment. "Lowering androgen levels or stopping them from getting into prostate cancer cells often makes prostate cancers shrink or grow more slowly for a time. *Bu, hormone therapy alone does not cure prostate cancer*," because, in time, the cancer becomes resistant to this treatment, according to the ACS, which adds, "Hormone therapy may control the cancer, often for a number of years, but it is not a cure. Usually, the cancer will change into a form that no longer needs testosterone to grow."[21] When the cancer no longer requires testosterone to grow, it is called androgen independent, or castration-resistant, and other treatments must be considered.

"Men with metastatic disease, stage IV disease, or those with high-risk disease who are undergoing radiotherapy as a primary treatment are typically good candidates for hormone therapy," says Dr. Evan Pisick, a medical oncologist, who practices in Chicago.

Hormone therapy may use a combination of medications that modify the body's hormone control system and cause the testes to stop making testosterone. This procedure replaces the earlier means of reducing testosterone through surgical castration, an orchiectomy, which has often had negative psychological effects. When castration is considered, the patient usually is given the option of having artificial testes implanted during his surgery for cosmetic and psychological purposes.

Currently, Lupron and Zoladex are two commonly used drugs in hormone therapy for prostate cancer. Anti-androgen blocks include the drugs (at the time of this writing) Eulexin, Casodex, and Nilandron. Yet another drug, DHT, is used in some cases. It is an androgen and, among other things, helps give males their male characteristics.

Another recent addition to the array of androgen depravation therapy (ADT) treatment options is Apalutamide (though still in phase 3 testing), which is specifically designed for men with nonmetastatic, castration-resistant (either chemical or physical) prostate cancer.

Significant results of a double-blind placebo-controlled phase 3 test showed that men taking Apalutamide maintained a metastasis-free life of 40.5 months versus 16.2 months for the men taking the placebo, according to a research report in the April 2018 issue of the *New England Journal of Medicine*.[22]

As we have noted earlier, and as pointed out in the *NEJM* report, "metastases are a major complication and [cause of] death among men with prostate cancer," therefore, achieving life-extension without metastasis is an important accomplishment.

The UCSF is optimistic about the effects of hormone therapy, positioning it in a positive light: "Working cooperatively with your partner to accommodate the changes resulting from hormone therapy and other treatments can help you remain sexually active. Various medications, as well as some mechanical methods, may help restore potency." However, the often-complete inability to attain an erection (impotence) is the result.

Potential short-term side effects include the following:

- Loss of desire for sex (libido)
- Itching
- Impaired sexual function
- Diarrhea
- Decreased muscle mass
- Weight gain
- Decreased mental capacity
- Mood swings
- Fatigue
- Hot flashes
- Depression
- Loss of body hair
- Nausea
- Insulin resistance
- Breast tenderness and breast growth
- Osteoporosis-caused bone fractures

A potential long-term side effect is that the patient's testosterone may not return to pretreatment testosterone levels.

All men who receive ADT will have some shrinkage of their testicles, and some will experience a total testicular disappearance, which may be more than a bit unnerving to some patients. The alternative perspective, physical castration, is much out-of-style today, but has its proponents and sound research supports their advocacy.

While chemical hormone deprivation is the currently preferred form of treatment, its predecessor—physical castration or bilateral orchiectomy—"has long been a mainstay of treatment for metastatic prostate cancer. However, due to concerns about cosmetic and psychological effects of surgical castration, that practice has been nearly eliminated in favor of medical castration," according to Cancer Therapy Advisor.[23]

However, "men who underwent surgical castration had significantly lower risks" of experiencing negative follow-on effects, as indicated by a ten-year study comprised of 3,295 men with metastatic prostate cancer, age sixty-six or older, and which lasted from January 1995 through December 2009. Within that group, 2,866 men were chemically treated, while 429 underwent bilateral orchiectomy.

For those men undergoing chemical treatment, there were six major adverse events:

1. Fractures
2. A blood clot that starts in a vein, venous thromboembolism
3. Peripheral arterial disease
4. Cardiac-related complications
5. Diabetes mellitus, related to how your body uses blood sugar
6. Cognitive disorders

In addition, patients' testosterone levels may not return to normal after completion of therapy.

Those men who underwent surgical castration, however, suffered "significantly lower risks of fractures, peripheral arterial disease, and cardiac-related complications than those (GnRH), the chemical alternative."

The men chemically treated for thirty-five months or more had an increased risk of the six new complications but achieved a three-year survival rate of 46 percent, compared to the lower survival rate of 39 percent for those who underwent surgical castration.

"I think these findings are important," said Dr. Quoc-Dien Trinh of Brigham and Women's Hospital and Dana-Farber Cancer Institute in Boston in an interview with Cancer Therapy Advisor. "Orchiectomy has almost disappeared as a treatment option for men requiring permanent testosterone blockade. I find it disconcerting that a perfectly reasonable, cost-effective surgical treatment with potentially less adverse effects and compliance issues than its pharmacologic equivalent has disappeared from medical practice for non-scientific reasons."

Despite the statistics, many men are understandably reluctant to be castrated, even with the promise of implantation of a testicular prosthesis, which mimics the appearance, look, and feel of testicles.

Intermittent Hormone Therapy

With intermittent hormone therapy—or intermittent androgen blockade—a patient receives the therapy dosage for a few months or over a year, with the expectation that the PSA will drop to zero or close to it. At that point, the dosing is stopped.

However, when the PSA rises, indicating the resumption of the body's production of testosterone, hormone therapy is resumed. As with the therapy itself, the length of time a patient stays off treatment may be from several months to over a year, according to the UCSF. Presently, there is no medical consensus as to the appropriate PSA level necessary to cease the treatment or the level to which it must rise to resume treatment. Studies to determine a range of suggested PSA levels are ongoing. The risks, physiological responses, and rates of rising and lowering of the PSA are also being studied.

Chemotherapy

Chemotherapy uses one or a combination of cancer-fighting drugs that are either injected into a vein or taken orally. The procedure may be recommended for patients with metastatic disease. Chemotherapy kills cancer cells, but also damages normal cells, and can cause significant side effects, which can seriously affect one's quality of life. Here's a partial list of the potential side effects:

- Diarrhea
- Loss of appetite
- Hair loss
- Mouth sores
- Nausea
- Vomiting

Active Surveillance

Active surveillance, or watchful waiting, may be recommended if:

- The cancer is very small, confined to one area of the prostate, and expected to grow very slowly.
- The patient is elderly, frail, or has other serious health problems that limit his life expectancy.[24]

The best candidates for this regimen are older men with small, low-grade cancers associated with low and stable PSA levels. Patients with a life expectancy greater than ten years may need a more aggressive approach.

Dr. Pisick, a CTCA medical oncologist near Chicago, says that he recommends active surveillance for 10 to 15 percent of his patients.

"Some of them may never need therapy due to low risk of their disease . . . while others may be too sick for therapy," he wrote.

In one UCSF Prostate Cancer Center study, about four hundred patients, in consultation with their doctors, chose active surveillance. Of that number, about 20 percent will receive treatment within two to three years after diagnosis, "after a change is detected such as a rapidly rising PSA level or increased tumor size." Those patients "have their PSA levels checked every three to four months, prostate ultrasounds every six to nine months, and prostate biopsies after one year of active surveillance, then again every one or two years."

Advantages of active surveillance are:

- No surgery involved
- No hospital stay
- No side effects such as urinary or fecal incontinence or erectile dysfunction
- Treatment delayed until the cancer begins to grow
- Less expensive than treatment.

Disadvantages of active surveillance are:

- Less proactive
- Frequent follow-ups with doctors for blood, rectal, and other tests
- Potential for repeat biopsies
- Potential for cancer to spread, or metastasize
- Potential for anxiety, worry, or other psychological stress

Clinical Trials

According to the UCSF, "Clinical trials primarily involve patients who have rising PSAs after treatment or who have more advanced, metastatic cancers." While new and trial treatments regularly emerge and are being tested on patients with new and recurrent cancers, "none of them are regarded as cures, or even as replacements for surgery, radiation or hormone therapy."[25]

These studies have three main phases.

1. Phase I studies involve a small number of patients and seek to assess safe and therapeutic dosages of a test drug.
2. Phase II trials involves more patients in an effort to determine if a new drug/dosage has benefits.
3. Phase III trials involve the largest groups of patients. One is the control group, which receives a standard therapy, and the second receives the new drug.

One good aspect of clinical trials is that "generally, patients being treated with these new approaches have experienced fewer side effects than patients receiving more traditional treatments."

Alternative Therapies

Alternative therapies include diet, nutrition and diet supplements, exercise, stress reduction, and various Asian medicines. The effectiveness of alternative therapies is unknown in the United States and, indeed, fall outside of the range of conventional treatments, with the exception of CyberKnife Image-Guided Therapy. Direct-to-consumer advertising about the CyberKnife procedure is believed to have created unrealistic expectations for the procedure as an option for treating prostate cancer patients. Such advertising began appearing in the New York City area in the spring of 2019 and "tends to emphasize benefits over risks and offer[s] unsubstantiated claims," cautioned Dr. Joseph Caputo, a urologist at both Columbia University Irving Medical Center and New York–Presbyterian Hospital.[26]

"That conclusion was made by investigators from Columbia University—after they created an online survey involving 400 men that used language lifted directly from an advertisement," according to *MedScape*. The results of the survey showed that, as a result of viewing the ad's claims, a significant percentage of men developed positive opinions about the CyberKnife procedure. Professional assessments of this form of cancer treatment, however, vary.

CyberKnife is an alternative to external radiation and deploys a "sophisticated system of delivering highly precise and focused radiation to tumors" in using real-time and is image-guided robotics.[27] Proponents say that CyberKnife is a noninvasive alternative to surgery that "can treat both cancerous and non-cancerous tumors anywhere in the body, including the brain, head and neck, kidney, liver, lung, pancreas, prostate and spine," according to Beth Israel Deaconess in Boston. The Boston hospital says that some of the improvements in the CyberKnife procedure include better quality of life for the following reasons:

- Performed as an outpatient procedure.
- Little to no recovery time or side effects.
- Virtually pain-free, with no sedation, incisions, or blood loss during treatment.
- Eliminates the risk of postsurgical complications.
- Shorter treatment compared to open surgery or traditional radiation therapy.

This technique may make it possible to treat cancers that cannot be treated using other techniques. It may also be an option for patients who cannot undergo surgery or seek an alternative to surgery.

IN OUR OPINION. . .

As we have learned so far in this book, the process of managing and surviving prostate cancer and its treatment, are no small challenges, require considerable personal courage, and will forever change your life. Therefore, managing your prostate cancer unquestionably should be approached with considerable respect, thoughtfulness, and a level of realism that is seldom required in daily decisions—at least, for many of us.

Indeed, both of us experienced some form of chemical treatment, and one of us specifically underwent Androgen Deprivation Therapy, or ADT. That experience perhaps illustrates one of the more dramatic validations of the phrase, "What you know may hurt you, but what you don't know can very well kill you."

I was not advised of some of the potential outcomes of my ADT treatment and was more than mildly surprised by one of them: I experienced severe testicular atrophy [shrinkage] to the point of total disappearance. I should have known that could happen, but I didn't. No one told me.

Furthermore,

Prostate cancer is a monumentally personal development in a man's life. The changes in his physical appearance—to say nothing about the major changes in his physical [read: sexual] abilities—can have enormous impact on how a man views himself, how he manages his own level of self-confidence, and how he deals with just about every aspect of his life.

Not taking these changes seriously and therefore not preparing a man for their onset is a big mistake, which may be fine in a test lab, but it certainly is not satisfactory in the real and humane world.

Indeed, we believe that doctors who deal with all forms of prostate cancer treatment too often tend to assume that their patients know—or will accept—the outcomes that have become commonplace to them but are drastic and dramatic for their individual patients. Therefore, we believe it is vital for patients undergoing prostate cancer treatment to ensure (through this book and other resources) that they know all of the possible outcomes that will result from their treatments, think about those outcomes, consider possible alternatives, and be prepared to physically and psychologically deal with the realities of their treatment.

The list of outcomes, a nice way of saying "changes," is relatively long and doesn't apply to all treatments, but some will apply to all, and all will apply to some treatments. Not to scare you, but here is a list of the personal physical changes (discussed further in later chapters) that can occur in your body and in your life:

- *Erectile dysfunction*
- *Urinary incontinence*
- *Fecal incontinence*
- *Testicular and/or penile reduction*
- *Painful hot flashes*
- *Change in emotions*
- *Nausea*
- *Loss of bone mass, osteoporosis-caused bone fractures*
- *Diarrhea*
- *Itching*
- *Weight gain*
- *Loss of body hair*
- *Breast tenderness*

- *Insulin resistance*
- *Depression that may abate or worsen*

Therefore, we believe that it is critically important to take prostate cancer and its many manifestations extremely seriously, and we also believe that the typical doctor-patient relationship must change. This is because of the special lifelong implications that prostate cancer treatment imposes on a patient, his spouse or partner, as well as others around him.

We also believe that doctors can no longer treat prostate cancer with the typical clinical (i.e., somewhat aloof) doctor-patient approach. The relationship must be team-oriented and should involve the following specialists:

- *The primary doctor*
- *Oncologist*
- *Urologist and other possible specialists*
- *A personal decision assistant familiar with prostate cancer treatment and outcomes*
- *The spouse or partner*
- *Possibly other family members*

We will deal further with these issues in section 4, "Managing My Prostate Cancer Decisions."

11

What About Metastatic Prostate Cancer?

Routine screening, or testing, can detect the presence of prostate cancer before it metastasizes. Once it does, there is characteristically no cure, just suppressive treatment.

Therefore, and despite the concerns of some prostate cancer professionals and varied recommendations from the USPSTF, there is a growing consensus among leading medical professionals that regular, cautious screening is necessary and valuable.

This is the case because once prostate cancer has been allowed to metastasize, treatment is generally only able to forestall the inevitable fatal end—if a man doesn't die from other causes first. And the path from metastatic detection to death is often very unpleasant.

Recent work by doctors at the Cleveland Clinic among men with very early-stage metastasized prostate cancer, however, has disproven the rule. In fact, some very early metastasis of limited scope can be cured; they are called "Oligometastatic Prostate Cancer."

In this chapter, however, we will assume that a man's prostate cancer was not detected—or treated—early enough to prevent it from fully metastasizing. Therefore, we will deal with the treatment for metastatic prostate cancer and the physical, functional, and psychological impacts of that treatment.

Prostate cancer that spreads to your bones does not become "bone cancer"; it remains prostate cancer, but it is prostate cancer that has invaded your bone structure, or some other organ. While your bones are often the first target of prostate cancer once it has escaped the prostate, it can spread into other organs, such as your liver, kidneys or lungs, or other locations. Currently, there is no cure for developed metastatic prostate cancer, so efforts to slow the cancer's growth and, if possible, contain

When prostate cancer expands outside of the prostate and gains access to the bloodstream, or metastasizes, it most commonly will reside in bones and other organs such as the liver, lungs, or brain. Bone metastases are seen in 85 percent to 90 percent of metastatic cases.

Source: "What Is Metastatic Prostate Cancer?" Prostate Cancer Foundation, accessed November 11, 2020, https://www.pcf.org/about-prostate-cancer/diagnosis-staging-prostate-cancer/prostate-cancer-metastases/.

it for the rest of a man's life are the available goals. As you will see, this has significant implications for the patient's quality of life until his death.

Since early-stage prostate cancer can be stopped if detected before it reaches advanced metastatic stages, it presents a very compelling argument for early, regular, and continued prostate testing. While such testing is critical, a rare and surprising situation arose for doctors at the Glickman Urological & Kidney Institute at the Cleveland Clinic in a patient with oligometastatic (limited and nearby) prostate cancer. Dr. Eric Klein described the incident this way:

"The patient had a high-grade prostate cancer invading nearby tissues as well as a nearby lymph node." The patient was "treated with hormone therapy for six months and then had his prostate and lymph node removed, followed by radiation to one metastatic site in the bone. Now eight years later, he has no cancer and isn't taking any medication for it."[1]

Dr. Klein wrote of his team's accomplishment: "If we can cure one patient with biopsy-proven metastatic prostate cancer in two sites, can we help other patients the same way? And even if we don't cure them, can we slow the cancer progression, so these patients live longer?" Based on that epiphany, the clinic is participating with other select medical centers recruiting for a clinical trial to see if the approach works consistently and more widely.

When metastatic prostate cancer is detected, its common early symptoms are:

- Bone pain
- Stiffness or deep pain in upper thighs, hips, or lower back

- Weight loss
- Fatigue
- Psychological changes such as depression

Late-stage metastatic prostate cancer generally implies a lack of responsiveness to treatment. Having migrated out of the prostate, late-stage metastatic prostate cancer generally spreads to the bones. The lack of response to treatment "may manifest as a rising PSA in a patient who was previously well controlled following surgery or radiation. Or, it may be a worsening of disease as evidenced on a CAT scan or other imaging test," according to Prostate.net.[2]

While early prostate cancer may go undetected because of its lack of symptoms, as it progresses—and metastasizes—men do experience symptoms. One note of caution, however, is that men should be aware that many of the symptoms of metastasized prostate cancer are also evidenced in BPH (benign prostatic hypertrophy) and prostatitis. BPH is a noncancerous enlargement of the prostate, and prostatitis is an inflammatory condition.

SIGNS OF METASTATIC PROSTATE CANCER

Advanced prostate cancer can have a significant impact on your lifestyle. Unfortunately, however, some men avoid talking about their symptoms, even with their doctors.

According to a Harris Poll commissioned by the International Prostate Cancer Coalition, "39% of the 410 men with advanced prostate cancer who were surveyed waited to tell their doctors about the symptoms they were experiencing, even though most of them realized the symptoms were associated with the cancer," according to the findings of the Prostate Cancer Symptoms Survey.[3] The men in the survey had cancer that had metastasized to the bones.

Their most common symptoms of advanced prostate cancer are the following:

- Fatigue, 85 percent—Excessive tiredness can be a symptom of the cancer, the treatment, or both.

- Pain in a specific area, 71 percent; generalized, 55 percent—The most common reason for pain in men with prostate cancer is bone pain. This pain typically develops slowly, so it's not uncommon for men to experience back pain. In most cases, the pain is described as aching, but it can be shooting and sharp. Infrequently, men experience bone fractures.
- Weakness, numbness, or difficulty walking, 55 percent—Men who experience this symptom typically have damage to the bones surrounding the spinal cord, which in turn affects the spinal nerves. This may lead to weakness or numbness in the legs. Pain associated with this condition is generally worse, but it differs from a patient's regular pain. There is also a chance that the impacted nerves may control urination and bowel movements.
- Poor sleep, 42 percent—Getting a cancer diagnosis is stressful, so you may not sleep well even if you are tired. Talk with your doctor, as there are medications or alternative therapies that may help with poor sleep.
- Trouble performing normal activities, 40 percent.
- Anxiety or distress because of pain, 40 percent.
- Constipation—This symptom is typically a side effect of medication taken to deal with pain rather than a symptom of advanced prostate cancer.
- Elevated calcium—If prostate cancer is in your bones, you can develop an elevated calcium level (hypercalcemia). Common symptoms include fatigue, increased thirst, and increased urination. Interestingly, a low calcium level, or hypocalcemia, is sometimes found but usually does not cause any symptoms. Hypocalcemia is usually a side effect of your advanced prostate cancer treatment.
- Loss of bladder and bowel functions—Known as urinary and fecal incontinence.
- Erectile dysfunction—Partial or complete impotence (inability to achieve an erection) is a possibility.

THERAPIES FOR ADVANCED PROSTATE CANCER

While the consensus holds that "there are no cures for advanced prostate cancer, but the disease can be controlled," men must take the disease quite seriously. The approaches generally taken include seeking to decrease the growth of the disease and minimize the pain experienced by the patient. Several ways to achieve these goals include the following.[4]

- Androgen deprivation therapy (ADT): This therapy targets the male hormones that that produce secondary sex characteristics (beard, body hair, muscle enlargement, deeper voice, sex drive, etc.). These hormones also stimulate prostate cancer growth. This process begins at puberty and continues throughout life.

  To reduce blood levels of testicular androgens, testicular activity can be blocked by drugs (medically) or by surgical removal of the testes (castration). To prevent cellular uptake of androgens from the adrenal glands, oral medication is given to block the androgen receptors on all cell surfaces. This combination of blocking both production and uptake of androgens is termed Androgen Deprivation Therapy.

  Surgical castration is irreversible, while the effects of ADT are gradual and sometimes may be reversed in the months after therapy is discontinued.

  ADT would be the perfect therapy for prostate cancer if not for the fact that most advanced prostate cancers gradually become resistant to ADT and are then called "castration resistant."
- Chemotherapy: Docetaxel and Cabazitaxel are chemotherapies that tend to prolong late-stage prostate cancer patients' lives. Docetaxel is usually combined with prednisone.
- Immunotherapy: In using immunotherapy certain cells that are unique to the cancer—but not the patient—can be targeted. This differentiates this therapy from other cancer treatments.
- PROVENGE: With this immunotherapy, a patient's "immune cells are harvested, modified to target and attack prostate cancer cells, and then infused back into the patient."
- Zytiga: Abiraterone acetate is an anti-androgen that inhibits the formation of testosterone, which is one of the hormones that causes growth of prostate cancer cells.
- Xofigo: Radium-Ra 223 dichloride is a radioactive injection used with bone metastases and when the prostate cancer is resistant to

medical or surgical treatments. It also seeks to lower testosterone levels.

- Xtandi: Enzalutamide is one of the few oral treatments for advanced, castration-resistant prostate cancer and works by slowing the growth of prostate cancer as it decreases its size.

Once the cancer has spread beyond the prostate, Androgen Deprivation Therapy (ADT) is the current "mainstay of treatment for metastatic prostate cancer."[5]

INCIDENCE OF METASTATIC PROSTATE CANCER RISING

The importance and urgency of metastatic prostate cancer research is evident in a Northwestern Medicine study, which shows that the number of new cases of metastatic prostate cancer climbed 72 percent in the decade from 2004 to 2013. "The report considers whether a recent trend of fewer men being screened may be contributing to the rise, or whether the disease has become more aggressive—or both," according to a report in the University's publication *Northwestern Now*.[6]

The Northwestern report states that the greatest increase in new cases of metastatic prostate cancer was among men fifty-five to sixty-nine years old, which rose 92 percent in the past decade. "This rise is particularly troubling because men in this age group are believed to benefit most from prostate cancer screening and early treatment."[7]

New independent research at Weill Cornell Medicine and New York Presbyterian Hospital has resulted in some confusion about increases in prostate cancer detection and any possible correlation with USPSTF recommendations issued in 2008 and 2012. (See our previous discussion about the USPSTF recommendations.)

The research used a national cancer database to identify 545,399 men over the age of forty who were diagnosed with prostate cancer between 2004 and 2013. Among men over age seventy-five, the researchers found that increases in both metastatic prostate cancer and aggressive nonmetastatic cancer had occurred since 2011, according to a report published in the December 29, 2016, edition of *JAMA Oncology*.[8]

Importantly, the researchers say their results show prostate cancer increases *may reflect the downstream effects of the USPSTF's recommendations* against routine PSA tests and underscore the need for healthcare policy leaders to reevaluate their approach to prostate cancer screenings.

"It's what most of us would have predicted, although somewhat sooner. There was a decrease in prostate cancer metastasis and death after the advent of PSA testing. Remove the screening and the rates of serious disease rise again," said lead author of the research report, Dr. Jim Hu, the Ronald P. Lynch Professor of Urologic Oncology at Weill Cornell Medicine and director of the LeFrak Center for Robotic Surgery at Presbyterian Weill Cornell Medical Center.

Dr. Hu conducted the study in collaboration with Dr. Art Sedrakyan, a professor of healthcare policy and research at Weill Cornell Medicine. They also examined data from a National Cancer Institute database (Surveillance, Epidemiology, and End Results Program), which tracks cancer incidence rates. "They found that the decline in PSA screening has significantly altered the way prostate cancer now presents, according to a Weill Cornell Medicine study."[9]

- 7.8 percent of men over seventy-five were diagnosed with metastatic prostate cancer in 2011, compared with 12 percent in 2013, an increase of 53 percent.
- The proportion of men diagnosed with "aggressive cancer" increased from 68.9 percent to 72 percent, an increase of 4.4 percent over the same period.
- There was no change in the rate of prostate cancer metastases among men under seventy-five years of age.

However, the results do not minimize the value of screening in younger men, according to Dr. Hu. This is because "the recommendation against PSA testing came later for younger men, so we might need to watch them over time" to see if they parallel with older men.

The results underscore the need to reevaluate PSA screening guidelines based on these data and reevaluation of prior screening trials that led to current PSA testing guidelines from the USPSTF, Dr. Hu said. "The public health message is that after years of decline, the incidence of metastatic disease has gone up," he continued, "And while the PSA test is not perfect, I don't think people should be told that this test has no value."

Dr. Hu emphasized that the implications of his study are that a man must have the "right to choose screening" to provide the opportunity for early diagnosis and treatment of prostate cancer. "The burden of over-treatment and side effects may no longer be sufficient to recommend against routine screening," Dr. Hu added.

IN OUR OPINION. . .

If for no other reason, the existence of metastatic prostate cancer should be sufficient reason for men to opt-in for early screening for prostate cancer—before it spreads and becomes incurable.

The results of Dr. Hu's research and the statistics provided by the National Cancer Institute as well as abundant other evidence clearly demonstrate the desirability of prostate cancer screening in order to halt the increase in prostate cancer that is already metastatic at the time of diagnosis.

This, of course, assumes that a man undergoing the prostate cancer screening and his physician and oncology team are cautious, prudent, and use enlightened discretion in interpreting all test results when choosing and timing of further procedures.

Of course, all medical decisions should be made with a similar level of caution.

Section 4

MANAGING MY PROSTATE
CANCER DECISIONS

12

Understanding Prostate Cancer's Emotional Impact

The onset and treatment of prostate cancer involves much more than the important job of trying to rid a body of the disease. It entails the nuanced vagaries of the human psyche and thus the relationship between a man and his mate and how he views himself in relationship to the world around him. Indeed, it directly has a significant impact on his very self-image.

To a large degree, today's medicine is very focused on treating the physical person, seeking to heal him and then to return him to productive life. While the not-so-subtle needs of a man's psyche are being increasingly recognized by medical professionals, that aspect of treating prostate cancer has yet to receive the level of attention it deserves and the appropriate integration into the treatment plan.

Understanding the emotional impact of prostate cancer is a complex task that melds the diverse demands of mind, body, and spirit. Of all the outcomes that can result from the treatment of prostate cancer, perhaps the most impactful is the one that medical professionals know the least about and have virtually no ability to treat: the unique relationship between a man and his mate and the emotional and physical bond that creates a unique understanding between them. That combination—and the man's image of himself—should be considered his "emotional aura." This aura reflects a man's ability to be the person he envisions himself to be. It is his perception of his own ability to effectively communicate affection and emotional sensitivity for and to his mate. This union is expressed by his capability to please—almost intuitively—the physical and emotional needs of one another. Because of his physiological changes and his diminished physical capabilities, however, it is not uncommon for prostate cancer patients to lose their ability to contribute proportionally to the emotional aura that they share with their mate. Because the prostate patient usually loses his ability to perform "normal" sexual functions once he enters the world of prostate cancer treatment, he must learn how to fill that physical void with a new expression of affection and connection with his mate. While out-reach and communicating affection may be an enhanced need during this time, the reality for prostate cancer patients may actually be the opposite, emotional withdrawal. This withdrawal not only has nega-tive implications for the man himself but also for his partner and, most importantly, for the strength of their relationship. Thus, they begin to lose the invisible emotional aura created by their bond over time.

In its most severe manifestation, this relationship-killer—prostate cancer—can lead to a dysfunction in the husband-wife union, which may result in dissolution of the marriage. Thus, prostate cancer will have ended the relationship for the parties without either one of them understanding exactly why that happened or their own lack of ability to recognize and overcome it.

This especially tragic outcome is one that many medical profession-als do not take responsibility for or help their patients cope with. The use of a professional counselor, including a personal decision assistant (PDA), is especially helpful in dealing with this problem. (The next chapter deals with the use of PDAs.)

This lack of knowledge—and therefore action—within the medical profession makes the condition all the more deserving of attention by a trained, sensitive, and practiced counselor. A PDA can be critical, even essential, in helping a couple maintain—or restore—the emotional aura that was an invisible but essential part of their relationship, which has now been replaced by:

- Sexual distance and termination of physical contact
- Emotional exclusion of the noncancer partner in private matters
- Denial of this emotional distancing
- Simple reduction in communication of all formal as well as inter-personal communication

Thus, the loss of the emotional aura creates a condition where two people who once shared their lives together are living in separate worlds, sharing a common house (not home) but little else. Despite the overwhelming importance of this aspect of prostate cancer treatment, it is an area that often receives little, if any, attention.

So, with that grim assessment of today's prostate cancer situation, it should be easy to understand the need for early identification of and appropriate support for maintaining that aura. In this way, the new needs of the prostate cancer patient and his spouse can be identified and met.

IN OUR OPINION. . .

We believe that the availability and intervention of professional counselors is essential for the stable recovery of many prostate cancer patients and the maintenance of his healthy relationship with his partner. We believe, too, that the emotional aura is in need of professional attention because:

1. *It cannot be identified by imaging, blood tests, or a doctor's examination.*
2. *American men have been reared to believe that they must withhold expressions of emotion, which may be viewed as signs of weakness.*
3. *No man is proud of becoming impotent, thus becoming a nonman.*

Newsweek *reported that "sex is one of the most universally uncomfortable topics of discussion," then quotes an American Cancer Society rehabilitation psychologist: "Sexuality is a very understudied area for the same reason it's an un-discussed area in clinical practice: People just don't want to talk about it—not in their research, not as a patient, not as a provider."[1] We believe that these social conditions conspire to create an enormous tragedy for many men and their spouses—as well as the relationship they created and once shared.*

13

Your Hidden Needs: Getting Insight and Help

"Shared decision-making represents the state-of-the-art in-patient counseling," according to ScienceDirect, *a publication from the Dutch publisher, Elsevier. As a result of the shared-decision-making process, patients have "greater knowledge and satisfaction as well as greater engagement" with their prostate cancer care.*

Elsevier further wrote this about shared decision-making: "Shared decision-making is an important component of high-quality health care delivery. . . . In appropriate circumstances urologists should adopt shared decision-making into routine clinical practice."[1]

However, as true as we believe these statements to be, the human and educational resources required to provide this level of high-quality shared decision-making and follow-on care seem to be limited in many situations.

Counseling and joint decision-making take two distinct forms at two very different times in a man's life when dealing with prostate cancer:

- *One is pretreatment, which is during the decision-making process.*
- *The second is postdiagnosis, during the critical and difficult accommodative period of treatment and the follow-on.*

Experience tells us that both are extremely important.

Doctors are often task oriented, however, which means that their goal is to treat a disease, cure it if possible, and move on to the next patient. So you might say that doctors have a fairly narrow field of vision that allows them to focus their special insights on purely medical issues for which they are trained.

While such a keen focus is an admirable trait in some circumstances, when dealing with prostate cancer, such single-mindedness may not accrue to the benefit of the whole patient. A patient's psychological health must be considered and managed at the same time he is tested for and treated for his physical prostate cancer.

Consistent with the traditional practice of medicine, Dr. Paul K. J. Han, at Maine Medical Center, Portland, and Tufts University School of Medicine, Boston, concluded that, "Most men in the US report little shared decision-making in prostate-specific antigen (PSA) screening, and the lack of shared decision-making is more prevalent in non-screened than in screened men."[2]

While a lack of shared decision-making may be a commonplace, it is less than ideal that a man would make such a decision about his health, indeed, his future quality of life without access to information about psychological outcomes. Needless to say, Dr. Han concluded that "Shared decision-making needs to be improved in decisions for and against PSA screening" and certainly in making choices about treatment.

Dr. Han's opinion was derived from a sample of 3,427 men ages fifty to seventy-four years old who participated in the 2010 National Health Interview Survey. They responded to questions on:

- The extent of shared decision-making, thus past physician-patient discussion of advantages, disadvantages, and scientific uncertainty associated with PSA screening.
- PSA screening intensity, that is, the number of tests in the past five years.
- The patient's socio-demographic and health-related characteristics.

The results are startling, though not particularly surprising:

- 64.3 percent of men reported "no shared decision-making," thus no physician-patient discussion of advantages, disadvantages, or scientific uncertainty.
- 27.8 percent reported "partial shared decision-making," thus physician-patient discussion of only one or two elements.
- 8.0 percent reported "full shared decision-making," thus discussion physician-patient discussion of all three elements.

In support of skilled decision-making, the American Urological Association (AUA) described the implications of the disease when it wrote: "The psychological impact of prostate cancer screening must be considered and viewed as a potential harm. . . . Along with the stress due to PSA screening and unnecessary biopsies, the diagnosis of prostate cancer alone may incite severe psychological stress."[3] Indeed, the AUA points to one study that shows "an increased rate of suicide and cardiovascular events" among men who are newly diagnosed with prostate cancer.

Not surprisingly, the AUA concludes that "potential harms must be carefully discussed" before a man begins a screening program. Further, at each step of a screening program, the patient should be given the information and the option of stopping treatment "based on his individual Quality of Life and longevity goals."

The simplest example is that, "for one man, the benefits of prostate cancer treatment may outweigh the risks. But, for another man with the same outcome probabilities, the risks may outweigh the benefits. In these "close call" situations, the AUA suggests that "a shared decision-making approach can be used to make the best possible decision about the intervention at the individual level."

A NEW, BROADER, AND IMPROVED APPROACH

Shared decision-making can have multiple benefits. For instance, the following can occur.

- The prostate cancer patient has time to "sound out" his reaction and feelings with an unemotional third party, the counselor.
- The patient can have an opportunity to "open up" to his partner or spouse with his innermost fears, emotions, and anxieties.
- The patient has time to consider the consequences of his decisions and anticipate how he might handle them, along with the benefits.

This shared-decision-making process can come in a number of forms.

- At one level, the patient and his doctor can candidly and thoroughly discuss procedures to be considered and the likely outcomes of those actions.

- At another level, the patient and his counselor (trained in prostate cancer procedures and outcomes) can discuss the risks and benefits.
- And on yet another level, after his procedures, the patient can consult with a psychologist (trained in handling prostate cancer cases) concerning the physiological changes a man undergoes and the emotions associated with those changes. These changes easily be associated with the patient's overwhelming loss of control.

Interventions, however, are not without risks, and the "net benefit of the intervention for an individual will depend on how a man (in the PSA context) values the possible outcomes," suggests the AUA.[4]

In the shared-decision-making process, "each choice has different patterns of outcomes, and the values a man places on those outcomes need to be considered in order to make an optimal decision. Such decisions are said to be 'preference sensitive,'" according to the article *Toward the Tipping Point* by Annette M. O'Connor in *Health Affairs*.[5]

"Preference-sensitive treatment decisions involve making value trade-offs between benefits and harms that should depend on informed patient choice," according to the School of Nursing at the University of Ottawa. "There is strong evidence that patient decision aids not only improve decision quality but also prevent the overuse of options that informed patients do not value."

In this shared-decision-making process, men should be able to involve a spouse, friend, or family member. However, the AUA suggests that, "It should not simply be assumed the man wants anyone else to participate." He may prefer to keep his condition and physical changes private. This information-sharing process can help the man and his partner or spouse understand the available options—and the risks and benefits of each option—while the patient can communicate his hopes, fears, and anxieties to the doctor and/or counselor.

Shared decision-making markedly contrasts with a more traditional and paternalistic approach to medicine in which knowledgeable doctors essentially tell men what they should do—suggestions that likely are based on the doctor's own values and preferences.

USING A COUNSELOR, WHEN AVAILABLE

While virtually all hospitals handle prostate cancer patients, not all hospitals have trained decision-making assistants on staff. To address this shortcoming, the International Patient Decision Aid Standards, or IPDAS-Collaboration, was created "to help men, and sometimes their families, determine the most suitable healthcare options and help patients clarify and communicate the personal value they associate with different features of their treatment options."[6]

By definition, personal decision assistants (PDAs) are individuals who have been trained and are equipped with the medical knowledge and professional communications tools needed to help men decide whether to proceed with prostate cancer screening and, if needed, treatment. They are not mere do-gooders who act as sounding boards for the patients but rather are individuals who have the personal ability, knowledge, and training to provide valuable assistance in assessing values and treatment outcomes with patients. The saying is that "knowledge is power," and one source of knowledge that gives prostate cancer patients power is the global organization Cochran Collaboration, whose goal is to provide independent information that enables better healthcare decisions. For the last twenty years, Cochran has provided high-quality information that has "transform[ed] the way health decisions are made." The global organization of more than thirty-seven thousand healthcare professionals in 130 countries gathers and summarizes research evidence with the goal of helping patients, professional caregivers, and decision aides make "informed choices about treatment." Cochran Collaborative produces "health information free of commercial sponsorship and other conflicts of interest."[7]

One of the many information services the Cochran Collaboration has made in recent years is to evaluate the shared-decision-making process using PDAs. The Collaboration identified eighty-six trials published through 2009 that involved over twenty thousand participants. Their analysis showed that using decision aides resulted in:

- Greater patient knowledge.
- More accurate risk perceptions when decision aides included probabilities.

- Decisions more consistent with values when explicit values clarification was available.
- Reduced decision-making conflict related to feeling uninformed and unclear about personal values.
- Fewer people who were passive in decision-making.
- Fewer people who remained undecided.

"Thus, there is strong evidence that a shared-decision-making process facilitated by PDAs improves the quality of preference-sensitive medical decisions," according to the AUA.[8] In addition to Cochran, the AUA's systematic review summarized the evidence supporting decision-making. Its high-quality evidence indicated that shared decision-making:

- Increased men's knowledge scores.
- Reduced decisional conflict.
- Promoted greater involvement in decision-making.

Information elements presented to men across shared-decision-making studies included the following:[9]

More commonly described issues:

- Presumed mortality benefit of screening in absolute terms
- Description of options after abnormal PSA is detected
- Likelihood of false-positive and false-negative results
- Description of subsequent tests needed for follow-up on abnormal screening results
- Harms of screening: additional procedures, hospitalization, life-threatening sepsis (septic shock in 0.1 percent to 0.3 percent of the cases treated)

Less commonly described but very important issues that should be discussed with a patient:

- Information about prostate gland anatomy and function
- Prostate cancer incidence and mortality
- Treatment options for early and late prostate cancer

- Complications of treatment options for early and late prostate cancer

That those four items fall into the "less commonly described" discussion area is tragic because they are four critically important issues. Men entering the long prostate cancer process should take note of these four issues and ensure that they are thoroughly discussed, or at least discussed to their complete satisfaction.

The panel concluded that PSA-based screening should not be performed in the absence of shared decision-making. Thus, as we have previously noted, the recommendation is against organized screenings in settings where shared decision-making is not part of routine practice, such as health fairs.

POSTPROCEDURE COUNSELING

While it seems that only modest attention is given by physicians and surgeons to pretreatment counseling and joint decision-making, it appears that even less attention is given to patients—and their families—in their adapting to the post-treatment changes.

The changes are often dramatic in a man's body and in his ability to function (such as urination and sexual performance). They have an impact not only on his emotional state but also have a potentially negative effect on his spouse or partner and on his relationship with others close to him.

While survivorship or mind/body medical programs may be available in some hospital situations, "It is indeed unfortunate that the overwhelming majority of cancer centers do not offer any comprehensive sexual rehabilitation programs," noted Dana-Farber Cancer Institute's (DFCI) Dr. Sharon Bober, who is an assistant professor of psychiatry at Harvard University and the founder and director of Dana-Farber's Sexual Health Program. "While there are growing numbers of programs for men and partners to help with the adaptive recovery process," Dr. Bober noted that "Sexual rehabilitation is still not readily accessible as part of the recovery process and that *men and their partners may have to advocate for themselves rather than rely on institutional guidance.*"

As evidence of this patient predicament, the majority of wives of men treated for prostate cancer reported "negative" or "very negative" impacts on their "sexual relationships" with their husbands, sometimes resulting in divorce.

Perhaps symptomatic of the casual attention given sexual recovery is the glib treatment given the subject by *Web*MD, which says simply, "If you and your partner have trouble with sexual or emotional closeness when you're in the middle of dealing with cancer, see a therapist for couples."[10]

The Cancer Treatment Centers of America (CTCA) has established what it calls a "mind-body medicine program" that is designed to support patients and their caregivers before, during and after cancer treatment. CTCA sees mind-body medicine as "an integral part of whole-person care" and "recognizes the powerful ways in which emotional, mental, social and behavioral factors may directly affect a patient's physical health."

Similarly, Boston's alliance of the Dana-Farber Cancer Institute with the Brigham and Women's Hospital for cancer treatment notes that, "Patients and their loved ones often face many new concerns and anxieties following a cancer diagnosis." The Dana-Farber Cancer Institute says that it offers a team of social workers, psychologists, psychiatrists, and other staff work available to work with patients, families, and other members of the healthcare team to provide integrated care and support for each patient's unique needs.[11] It focuses on five specific areas of patient intellectual and emotional assistance:

- Social work
- Support groups
- Adult psychosocial oncology
- Pediatric psychosocial oncology
- Spiritual care

DFCI claims that it will "work closely with your oncologist, nurses, and other members of your care team to ensure that the care you receive is both comprehensive and coordinated." Despite that, there is little evidence of any integrated effort along these lines of a mind-body experience—other than pamphlets lying about on waiting room end tables.

Similarly, CTCA says that in its counseling programs, "licensed mental health and allied professionals offer caring relationships and therapeutic practices and techniques" to help prostate (and other) cancer patients and their caregivers respond to a cancer diagnosis and treatment. The center also instructs them on methods of reducing stress "so you are better able to improve your health, relationships and overall well-being."

The center further explains that its "licensed mind-body therapists conduct prostate cancer support groups, provide counseling for patients and their partners, and help them get clear answers to their medical questions from the oncology team."

Further integration of the psychological aspect of the healing process—from before treatment through the aftershocks—is used at the University of Michigan. There, Daniella Wittman, a social worker and certified sex therapist at the Rogel Cancer Center, provides strategies for how couples can renew their sex lives following prostate cancer surgery. The perceived importance of Wittmann's work is recognized by the fact that she is imbedded in the Urology Department, and patients get access to an extensive level of behavioral information both before and after prostate cancer treatment. In many circles, the Rogel approach to patient interaction and support serves as a national model that deserves emulation.

In some cases, however, patients are pretty much on their own. As one such nationally recognized hospital in Florida writes on its website, "When you receive a diagnosis of prostate cancer, you may experience a range of feelings—including disbelief, fear, anger, anxiety and depression. With time, each person finds his own way of coping with a prostate cancer diagnosis."[12]

By contrast, the medical center at the University of California at San Francisco addresses what they call "Psycho-Oncology" in this way:

> Our team works closely with other cancer center providers to identify and address psychological and social distress, including the stresses of illness and medical treatment and concerns with relationships and caregiving. We also help patients learn behavioral strategies for coping with pain, insomnia, challenges with eating and other issues. We teach goal setting and mind-body strategies to help patients make meaningful changes that improve their quality of life, regardless of their diagnosis.[13]

IN OUR OPINION. . .

Prostate cancer counseling, and simple education, are necessary and important parts of the experience of working with your doctor.

At this time, when decisions have "forever consequences," many men deal with prostate cancer issues as a virtual illiterate, yet this ignorance concerns what will be some of the most important decisions of their lives. At the same time, a prostate cancer patient's spouse or partner should be included in the counseling and education processes because their life also will be materially impacted.

Leaving a stack of brochures on a waiting-room table about some form of decision-making help is good, but quite inadequate. This is a time of incredibly important decision-making, and rather than be left to chance, it should be organized and thoughtful.

As Omar Khayyam wrote in the Rubaiyat:
"The moving finger writes; and, having writ, moves on."
There are no redos.
This is it.

14

Prostate Cancer Realities Are Different Than You Think

Prostate cancer patients seem to have two problems in common.

- *Their expectations of the impact on their sexual and functional lives are much more positive than the reality they will experience.*
- *This mismatch between their expectations and the real world often results from inadequate preoperative counseling.*

As a result of this disconnect between perception and reality, the results of prostate cancer treatment can be disappointing. These results can have negative long-term effects on one's self-image and his relationship with his partner, and others around him.

Unfortunately, research shows that positive treatment outcome expectations often exceed actual outcomes. Some facilities utilize a true team approach that may commence well before surgery begins. The goal is to convey an appreciation for the realities and magnitude of what is about to take place. Ideally, the team approach will continue after the physical treatment—such as surgery—and through the recovery period.

After cancer treatment ends, patients expect life to return to normal. What they often find, however, is that "normal" means something quite different than it did before cancer, according to Daniela Wittman, a social worker and certified sex therapist at the University of Michigan's Department of Urology in Ann Arbor.[1] Any prostate cancer patient who enters a treatment regime with such an out-of-focus perception of what "normal" will be like after treatment has either not been fully informed by his medical team or has not fully listened to what that team told him about his impending treatment.

Ms. Wittmann explains that "asking for help in sexual matters is not easy for either the person who asks or for the person from whom help is sought. Most people consider sexual activity a private matter and feel awkward when discussing sexual difficulties, even within the couple. In a provider-patient relationship, the dynamics of help-seeking can be burdensome, if one or both members of the partnership feel uncomfortable broaching the subject."

This uncomfortable situation is particularly troublesome since "more than half of men undergoing radical prostatectomy have unrealistic expectations about some of the outcomes," writes MedPage Today, which cites Ms. Wittmann and her colleagues at Michigan's Rogel Cancer Center for some amazing statistics about sexual function and urinary incontinence.[2] One year after prostate surgery, for example, 61 percent of men expected the same or better sexual function, whereas 60 percent of men expected difficulties with urinary incontinence to be the same or better.

The statistics were the result of questionnaires completed by patients before treatment and one-year after undergoing radical prostatectomy. Called the *Expanded Prostate Index Composite Questionnaire*, the goals were "to get a picture of their urinary, bowel, hormonal and sexual function[s]" before surgery and a year later. Astonishingly, Wittmann and her colleagues found that a substantial proportion of patients—17 percent for sexual function and 12 percent for incontinence—expected better performance a year after surgery than before the procedure, despite the fact that patients had been counseled that such outcomes were not at all likely.

Obviously, the "message of prostate surgery results [are] not getting through. More than half of men undergoing radical prostatectomy have unrealistic expectations about some of the outcomes," according to Michael Smith, a North American correspondent for MedPage Today.[3]

The alarming nature of these finding suggests that preoperative education is either inadequate or not internalized by patients. These statistics strongly argue in favor of postop education and counseling by trained professionals.

Analysis of the 152 participants showed:

- 36 percent and 40 percent expected the same personal performance relative to their urinary incontinence and sexual function, respectively, while 12 percent and 17 percent expected better function.

- 47 percent and 44 percent of patients had lower than expected function for urinary incontinence and sexual function, respectively.
- For "urinary irrigative symptoms," expectations matched or were better than outcomes for 78 percent of patients.

For bowel and hormonal functions, expectations matched outcomes 92 percent and 86 percent, respectively, having outcomes that were the same as or better than expected. "The differences may arise from the way pre-op counseling is given," Wittmann said. Researchers cautioned, however, that the questionnaire's response rate was low: 152 out of 526. They also noted that the counseling on sexual matters was standardized, while information provided by surgeons on other outcomes was not standardized.[4] "If you understand the physical and sexual side effects that you could have during or after prostate cancer treatment, you'll be better prepared to handle them," as *Web*MD correctly points out.[5]

Regardless of what a man thinks his sexual and functional outcome may be, the realities speak for themselves. A man's prostate cancer treatment negatively affects a couple's sexual relationships in seven out of ten instances, according to women polled in a study led by Dr. Scott Ramsey of the Public Health Sciences Division at Fred Hutchinson Cancer Research Center in Seattle, as reported in the *Journal of Sexual Medicine*.[6]

In Dr. Ramsey's study, researchers followed eighty-eight prostate cancer patients and their female partners for up to a year after treatment. At the six-month mark,

- 39 percent of the partners reported a "somewhat negative" effect on their sexual relationship.
- 12 percent reported a "very negative" effect.

At the twelve-month mark, the percentage of partners who found that cancer treatment had produced a "very negative" impact on their sexual relationship more than doubled, probably due to the delayed effects of radiation therapy.

Similar results come from a study that evaluated sexual functions of men at nine academic medical centers, according to Dr. Martin G. Sanda, the director of the prostate care center when he was associated with the Beth Israel Deaconess Medical Center in Boston. He is now a professor of urology and chair at Atlanta's Emory University School of Medicine.

Overall, 35 percent of men in the surgery group, 37 percent of men in the radiation group, and 43 percent of men in the brachytherapy (seeds) group were able to have sexual intercourse two years after treatment.[7] Since the statistics reported are for those men who *were* able to have sexual intercourse, we are left to the conclusion that the majority of men in each of the three treatment categories were *unable* to achieve sexual intercourse. (Since the study followed the men for only two years, it is not considered definitive; however, the results produced are consistent with finding in longer-term evaluations.)

Medical and psychiatric social worker Rick Redner, who graduated from Michigan State University, lists "8 Reasons Why Sexual Desire Is Reduced After Prostate Surgery."[8] While his list is far from exhaustive, we present it below in an abbreviated form. (His August 4, 2017, article appears at this link in the online publication *Prostate Cancer News Today*.)

1. Coping with cancer can create fear and anxiety that "can impact sexual desire."
2. Depression "leads to a noticeable reduction in desire or interest in sex."
3. Losing urinary control at any time "may greatly impact a man's desire for sex."
4. Climacturia is leaking or urinating during organism, which may cause a couple to avoid sex altogether." However, "few, if any, men are told it's possible" before treatment.
5. Loss of ejaculation "can affect the pleasure men feel."
6. Change in orgasms and painful orgasms that "significantly reduced intensity and pleasure" make orgasms less desirable, and painful orgasms activate "a built-in desire to avoid pain."
7. Reduction in penis size, which may "cause some degree of shame that will greatly impact a man's interest in sex."

8. Erectile dysfunction, or the inability to achieve an erection, "can have a devastating impact on a man's libido and desire for all forms of physical contact."

From a purely clinical perspective, a successful return to "normal" sexual performance depends on a variety of factors that include a man's age, the past strength of his erections, and the degree to which his surgeon was able to spare nerves surrounding the prostate, according to Michigan's sex therapist, Ms. Wittmann.

While erectile dysfunction is among the most common long-term side effects of prostate cancer surgery, treatments are available to remedy the dysfunction—but with varying degrees of restorative success. If your surgeon was not able to accomplish sufficient nerve sparing, according to Wittmann, supplemental aids such as a vacuum pump, penile injections and suppositories, and penile implants are also possibilities.

In addition to surgery, *Web*MD states that chemotherapy and hormone therapy can cause weight gain, a lowered libido, fatigue, and urinary incontinence.

IN OUR OPINION. . .

We believe that having read this far, you will readily understand why we are concerned about the misalignment between prostate cancer patients' expectations (or lack thereof) for their conditions and abilities after treatment and the realities they will actually experience. You could say that this is a case of "Just because you say it isn't so, doesn't make it go away."

Even so, we believe that a loss of sexual initiative can be due to many factors, such as Mr. Redner's list of eight we just stated. But, as with many things in life, when we know what to expect during and after an experience, the more accepting we are of the subsequent ups and downs.

We don't believe, however, that sufficient emphasis has been given to the need to inform patients of what they will likely—or assuredly—experience following their prostate cancer treatments.

15

Adjusting: The Question of Intimacy

Prostate cancer is problematic, at best. While a man and his partner or spouse must deal with the disease, treatments, and side effects, the ultimate impact is on the closeness a man has with his spouse or partner. That may be the most devastating change.

Considerable courage is required to deal with the progression—and possible remission—of the disease; however, no small amount of courage also is required to manage the emotional impacts of the disease on a man, his spouse or partner, and their relationship.

While it is not uncommon for women to discuss among themselves the implications of breast cancer on their bodies and their relationships, the reality among men is quite different. Men simply don't talk about sex—except in an occasional locker room fashion—and that silence is not helpful when prostate cancer arises.

Let us quote Newsweek, *which we cited a bit earlier in this book, but which is worth citing again:*

"Sex is one of the most universally uncomfortable topics of discussion. . . . And sexuality is a very understudied area for the same reason it's an un-discussed area in clinical practice: People just don't want to talk about it—not in their research, not as a patient, not as a provider."[1]

Surviving prostate cancer requires physical *and* emotional strength; regardless of how you look at it, there is nothing simple or easy about the experience. The issues of sex and intimacy—which are quite different subjects—are paramount in this process.

Both areas, "connectedness" and "sex," are problematic and present "enormously frustrating and humiliating" opportunities for couples after prostate cancer treatment, as one Seattle survivor testifies. When Chris Pearce was diagnosed with prostate cancer about eight years ago, memories of his father, who had died from complications of the disease, flashed through his head. While Pearce's first priority was getting the care he needed, he also worried about the impact on sexual function his father faced after treatment. "I was very keen on not getting the same side effects," Pearce recalled.

Pearce chose a nerve-sparing robotic prostatectomy to help preserve his sexual ability, but within a year, his PSA levels began to rise, and he received radiation treatment at Seattle Cancer Care Alliance. "I was delighted to be finished with my treatment, but my worst point was after the radiation. I took Viagra and things like that, but it didn't help," said Pearce, a fifty-eight-year-old engineer.

At the time he was in a marriage that was winding down, and the sexual side effects from treatment added pressure. "It was enormously frustrating and humiliating for me," he said.[2] "I also found myself getting increasingly angry over the most trivial and stupid things."

It's an issue often faced by many of the estimated quarter of a million US men diagnosed each year with prostate cancer—and their spouses and partners. While no one is ever prepared for a diagnosis of cancer, "the diagnosis of prostate cancer is especially agonizing," says Rhonda Fine, a PhD, and board-certified sex therapist at the American Academy of Sexologists. When this diagnosis occurs, there is a "vast array of emotions that come into play. Extreme sadness, fear and grief are at the core."

Dr. Fine and others believe that "the integrity of a couple's relationship before prostate cancer is a key indicator of how the couple will deal with the impact of cancer." She suggests that "Silence is a powerful enemy. Good communication enables one the freedom to share their feelings, fears and emotions," and very importantly, "It eliminates mind reading." "Intimacy cannot exist without effective communication," Dr. Fine says. "It gives one a sense of security. It is intimacy, which will nourish the relationship during stressful times. Intimacy gives the relationship the quality of togetherness and camaraderie, acceptance and validation by one's partner. which foster the feeling of 'being alive.'"

While the man personally must deal with and manage the diagnosis, treatment, and their outcomes, his partner plays a significant role in providing "support emotionally, physically and socially" throughout that process. Dealing with the impact prostate cancer treatment has on intimacy does not occur in isolation. And intimacy, of course, has its physical manifestations as well as emotional.

Perhaps a revealing insight into this situation of intimacy and sex is the old line that, "Women use sex to get intimacy; men use intimacy to get sex." As one expert doctor wrote, intimacy is about connectedness and sharing of a deeper bond, which that transcends sexual activity. That observation comes from Dr. Don S. Dizon, director of Women's Cancers at Lifespan Cancer Institute, director of Medical Oncology at Rhode Island Hospital, and a professor of medicine at the Warren Alpert Medical School of Brown University.

Dr. Dizon asked a group of men recovering from prostate cancer surgery, "What do you mean by intimacy?" One hesitant attendee responded: "Intimacy is holding my wife's hand. It's being able to kiss her and not feel shy or embarrassed that I cannot have an erection. It's lying in bed, just holding her. I think it's not about sex, at least for me."[3] Dr. Dizon and other professionals believe that "sexual intimacy goes beyond the ability to have an erection or vaginal intercourse. It [has] to do with lingering hugs, touching and communication."

However, an array of emotions and anxieties play a powerful role in a man's self-confidence in approaching intercourse—and successfully accomplishing it—and satisfying his partner. Eight "reasons" why men lose their sex drive after their prostate is removed may include the following:

1. Anxiety: Coping with cancer produces fears and anxieties that can produce real physical changes and have a negative impact on a man's sex drive.
2. Depression: Depression is a common postsurgical emotion, and men express their depression much differently than women. Men often exhibit this emotion through a loss of energy, a loss of interest in previously enjoyed activities, and a loss of interest in sex. Women, on the other hand, typically become sad.
3. Loss of urinary control: The loss of urinary control can occur at any time during the day or night and will require the use of absorbent pads to control the leakage. Loss of urinary control is a common side effect of prostate surgery, and it may negatively affect a man's desire for sex.

4. Climacturia: This medical term simply means urinary leaking during sexual contact or orgasm. This is another medical shortcoming that few men are warned about before treatment, and when it appears, it can be a complete "turn-off" for a man and/or his partner or spouse.
5. Loss of ejaculation: Men lose their ejaculation ability after prostate cancer surgery. This can cause a feeling of sadness or a sense of loss after orgasm; therefore, some men may avoid intercourse altogether.
6. Reduced intensity or painful orgasm: Some men experience a loss of intensity of their orgasm or experience painful organisms. Since our natural tendency is to avoid pain, this can translate into avoiding sexual contact.
7. Reduced penis size: Some men report a reduced penis size, which is embarrassing, and may result in their avoiding sexual activity.
8. Erectile Dysfunction: After prostate cancer surgery, most men will experience an inability to achieve an erection. This can result in a devastating impact on a man's sex drive and even his willingness to have physical contact.

The hush-hush nature of sexual practices and medical treatment of sexual problems like prostate cancer exacerbate the difficulties men experience in dealing with the disease. While sex is different than intimacy, genuinely valid sexual relations are seldom possible without the trust that comes with intimacy. And it is these elements of true intimacy that are often absent in relationships. Because of the confusion between sex and intimacy, researching the broad subject is not easy.

Sex is perhaps the most universal of subjects but is virtually ignored except at times of distress—like when a man experiences the onset of prostate cancer. Because of these problems dealing with sex, creating an environment of intimacy is difficult, despite the fact that such a condition is especially meaningful for the man seeking to recover from prostate cancer. The disconnect between sex and intimacy tests the very core of a couple's relationship. Intimacy may be considered the most valuable glue in holding together a positive spousal relationship after the development of prostate cancer.

If one assumes that interpersonal intimacy existed before the prostate cancer, then a Harvard Medical School paper on "prostate cancer and relationships" is correct to state that, "re-establishing intimacy after treatment requires honest communication about each person's needs."[4] If interpersonal intimacy was not on a solid foundation before the prostate cancer process, then it likely will not emerge after the discovery of prostate cancer.

Thus, the Harvard paper states, "a therapist can help start the conversation," especially when the assistance begins early in the treatment process; however, the therapist cannot create what did not exist before treatment began.

Yet, it is possible even for doctors to have epiphanies, as was the case for Dr. Dizon, who "had done so much research about the physical aspects of male sexuality [that he] had not given much thought about intimacy, relationships and the psycho-emotional aspect" of the male-female relationship.

For Dr. Dizon, among the research papers that he favors is one that describes the "three-factor solution that conceptually encompassed perspectives on intimacy and sexuality."

Factor 1 [is] the importance of communication, emphasizing the importance of acknowledging that there are a range of sexual and intimate practices available to patients and their partners post-cancer.

Factor 2 involves the normalization of the sexual experience across the journey with cancer, requiring re-negotiation of what these mean to patients and their partners, and seeking ways to evolve alternative sexual practices.

Factor 3 emphasizes the importance of intimacy, even for patients where actual physical sexual relations may not be wanted, desired, or even possible.[5]

THE VERY PERSONAL SIDE OF INTIMACY

A truism accepted by most prostate cancer recovery professionals is that real intimacy goes well beyond sexual intercourse; it is a mental connection, an almost intuitive ability to communicate with another person. This unique closeness is often enhanced as one approaches the final days and can be aided by effective and thoughtful palliative care.

The following commentary, entitled "At Life's End, The Gift Of Intimacy," aired on May 14, 2019, on Boston's WBUR-FM on the regular program called *Cognoscenti*.[6] It was presented by Dr. Ashwini C. Bapata, a palliative care physician at Boston's Massachusetts General Hospital and a Harvard Medical School instructor.

I met Charles, a self-proclaimed foodie, while he was being treated for esophageal cancer. The tumor had narrowed his esophagus, making it hard to enjoy his chipotle-rubbed steaks. He had lost 30 pounds in a few months and had constant throat pain and nausea.

As his palliative care doctor, I helped make his pain and nausea tolerable. . . . Unfortunately, his cancer progressed despite aggressive treatment. He no longer had the strength to work or drive. He stopped gardening because he didn't have the stamina to kneel, dig and sow seeds. His hikes through the woods became traipses around the house with a walker.

I often ask my patients with life-threatening illness to define their goals. What would be most important to them if time were short? Charles's answer was emphatic.

"I don't want to be a burden to my wife," he said. "If I can't eat or poop or get out of bed, use the morphine drip. Let me go." Many patients tell me something very similar. It's as though the possibility of dependence is harder to cope with than the possibility of dying.

As the cancer spread, it limited Charles to eating only pureed food. Then he needed a commode placed next to his bed. Eventually, he was completely bedridden and very thin, barely a lump under the covers. One day, during a home visit, I stood at the bedroom threshold, watching his wife Ellen grab a diaper, slide it under the soiled one, clean Charles with wet wipes. She chucked the soiled diaper in the trash and combed her fingertips through his wispy hair. This was exactly what Charles didn't want—lingering like an unwanted guest in his own home.

As a palliative care doctor, I have learned it is the lucky few who drive themselves to work one day, and then die peacefully in their sleep that night. For most people, dying is some version of Charles' experience. For some cancer patients, like Charles, the change is rapid.

During the home visit, Ellen pulled me aside and shared her struggles. She had not been sleeping. She drifted in the shallows of sleep, surfacing frequently to scan the baby monitor for moaning or grimacing, signs that Charles needed more pain medications. During the two hours each day when the home health aide watched Charles, she rushed from the grocery store to the pharmacy and then to the bank, before speeding home to ward off an impending crisis.

Ellen told me that despite her exhaustion and sadness, there was still intimacy. For Ellen and Charles, this was the most uninterrupted time they'd had together since the birth of their children nearly half a century ago. Those early mornings once defined by ironing collared shirts, hissing tea kettles and clamoring kids were a distant memory. These mornings, she perches on her overstuffed armchair spoon-feeding Charles his favorite homemade vanilla custard. When he is done, she dabs his mouth clean, and then reclines in her chair, turning her attention to the muted morning TV show. His bony fingers search till they find hers, and the two doze off together. I frequently find them together like this, their hands entwined.

These moments are not unique to Ellen and Charles. I have witnessed them among so many of my patients. On afternoon rounds I saw a woman cuddling in the hospital bed with her husband, her legs enveloped by his.

Like Charlie, many patients have told me that depending on others is unacceptable. Yet, in witnessing these moments, I can't help but think that even in those last days and weeks of life, there are opportunities for intimacy, for affirmation, and for love—parting gifts shared with those who will continue to live. Perhaps the period of dependence exists for the possibility of these valuable moments.

IN OUR OPINION. . .

"Intimacy cannot exist without effective communication," Dr. Rhonda Fine states in His Prostate Cancer. "It gives one a sense of security. It is intimacy, which will nourish the relationship during stressful times. Intimacy gives the relationship the quality of togetherness and camaraderie, acceptance and validation by one's partner, which fosters the feeling of 'being alive.'"

Unfortunately, in some countries (notably the United States), sex has become confused with closeness and intimacy, which does not auger well for the prostate cancer patient.

Further complicating a man's recovery from prostate surgery is the possibility that solid, open communications between the man and his partner or spouse did not exist even before his treatment. If that is the case, the process of sexual recovery after treatment is manifestly more difficult.

A Correct and Expansive View of Palliative Care

Palliative care is often, and mistakenly, associated with the end-of-life and hospice care. Because of this unfortunate and erroneous association, the palliative care treatment option is sometimes overlooked during the earlier stages of prostate cancer, and therefore many men do not benefit from this effective and unique form of care.

This is unfortunate, because the negative physiological and psychological effects of prostate cancer—and its treatment—can be reduced at any stage through the effective application of palliative care. Fortunately, though, multidisciplinary palliative care teams are being formed throughout the United States and in other parts of the world.

Palliative care is designed to sooth and comfort a patient as opposed to curing his disease, which seeks to eliminate or reduce the cause of pain. Therefore, it is often associated with end-of-life care, which may be one reason that it "is under-utilized for prostate cancer despite evidence showing benefit in several patient populations," according to the World Health Organization (WHO).[1]

"Despite significant advances in understanding the benefits of early integration of palliative care with disease management, many people living with a chronic life-threatening illness either do not receive any palliative care service or receive services only in the last phase of their illness," according to Dr. Pippa Hawley, a Canadian who has worked among Pacific peoples in need of palliative care. In her article, "Barriers to Access to Palliative Care," Dr. Hawley wrote that she explains to professionals the reasons for failure to provide palliative care in the hopes that her recommendations will help overcome palliative care barriers.[2] She also emphasizes the importance of providing palliative care accurately.

To better understand the true meaning of the term, she added, "Palliative care can be described briefly as a way of caring for people with life-threatening illnesses which focuses on quality of life, which . . . addresses patient needs in the physical, social, psychological, and spiritual domains:

1. Meticulous prevention and management of symptoms, including pain.
2. Excellence in communication, in discussion of goals of care and advance care planning.
3. An extra layer of support for practical needs, particularly with respect to care provided at the patient's home."

The American Society of Clinical Oncology agrees, emphasizing that, "Experts warn that dismantling this [end-of-life] misconception is critical to the early integration and effectiveness of palliative care in [the prostate cancer] patient population."

Dr. Christopher Kane at the University of California San Diego also emphasizes the unfortunate outcomes resulting from a linkage of palliative care with end-of-life care and maintains that the inappropriate connection "is not helping patients." Unfortunately, he continues,

Many patients can benefit from palliative care early in the course of disease management because palliative care specialists have an expertise in symptom management. . . . If the patient's symptoms are well controlled, they are more likely to continue with effective treatment. Palliative care should be initiated at the same time as treatment; and doing so does not mean that there will necessarily be a change in the intensity or objective of that treatment, which needs to be communicated to patients.

When palliative care is provided, it ideally involves a team approach. Those team members seek to improve a patient's quality of life and to make his daily activities more comfortable by easing pain and other problems associated with your treatment. The focus is not only on a patient's physical symptoms but also on his emotional and psychological well-being. Indeed, psychological care and counseling may be at least as important as treating physical aspects of prostate cancer. While palliative care is often associated with an end-of-life function of hospice care, the fact is that palliative care can begin at any stage of your disease. Any medical professional can provide palliative care, but many hospitals provide specialists to provide the services.

Oncology guidelines suggest initiating palliative care "early in the course of illness in conjunction with other therapies that are intended to prolong life, including chemotherapy and radiation," according to the WHO.[3] In fact, "One of the most important goals of palliative care is easing the physical symptoms of the cancer itself and any side effects from treatment," according to *Web*MD.[4] These services can be provided to help a patient understand and manage a range of prostate cancer and treatment problems ranging from urination, erectile and ejaculatory dysfunction, and bone pain that may be associated with certain types of treatments or drugs.

Fatigue is a common side effect of many prostate cancer treatments, and a palliative care specialist can recommend changes in lifestyle that will increase the patient's energy. In consultation with your doctor, the palliative specialist may also suggest a change of drugs. Dietary changes and some forms of physical therapy may ease problems with nausea, vomiting, breathing, sleeping, and appetite.

While it may seem strange, according to *Web*MD, "Sometimes chemotherapy, radiation therapy, and surgery may be considered 'palliative' care because they do ease pain by shrinking tumors," even if they do not provide a cure.

Palliative care experts and prostate cancer support groups can help with management of psychological problems including depression, anxiety, and fear. Hospital chaplains and other palliative care professionals can discuss spiritual or religious issues.

Since effectiveness of prostate cancer treatment has advanced over time, men can live with symptoms for longer periods. Therefore, interdisciplinary palliative care teams—which may include physicians, nurses, social workers, chaplains, pharmacists, psychologists, physical therapists, and nutritionists—focus on symptom management. This helps maintain an acceptable quality of life, which is especially important since extended life spans naturally increase the duration of potential discomfort a man may experience.

As the prostate cancer progresses, so does the importance of palliation, because the progression of the disease results in such complications as bony metastases, spinal cord compression, lymphedema, and urinary obstruction. In addition, treatment often causes fatigue and anemia. Significant psychological effects may include depression, anxiety, poor coping ability, altered view of self and the future, lack of empowerment, and disrupted partner intimacy, according to *Translational Andrology and Urology,* which states that the beneficial aspects of palliative care can be especially valuable in at least three treatment circumstances.[5]

1. Localized treatment with surgery and/or radiation may cause the following conditions:

   - Pain
   - Fatigue
   - Incontinence
   - Diarrhea
   - Gross hematuria
   - Erectile dysfunction
   - Bowel dysfunction
   - Urethral stricture development

2. A biochemical recurrence after localized therapy among men with regional or metastatic disease may be treated with androgen deprivation, which may cause the following conditions:

   - Nausea
   - Immune suppression
   - Vomiting
   - Psychiatric effects
   - Diarrhea
   - Weight gain
   - Hot flashes
   - Myalgias
   - Loss of libido
   - Osteoporosis
   - Insomnia
   - Gastric ulceration
   - Gynecomastia, male breast swelling
   - Lower urinary tract symptoms

3. Novel therapies for incurable prostate cancer include chemotherapies, targeted-hormonal therapies, and immunotherapies, which
   may prolong survival for a few months but may also result in
   severe side effects such as those previously mentioned.

The case in favor of early palliative care is succinctly made in the
American Journal of Managed Care, which states that, "Cancer patients
[who] receive palliative care earlier in their treatment demonstrate
higher satisfaction, better symptom management, and an increased
survival rate."

IN OUR OPINION. . .

*A major disservice is imposed on men with prostate cancer based on the
belief that palliative care is either a part of hospice care or the same
as hospice care. However, palliative care clearly is a discipline unto
itself and an important one for prostate cancer patients; it should not
be confused with hospice care even though it may be conjoined with it.*

*Another misconception—even among medical professionals who
treat and manage cancer cases—is that palliative care and its administering teams are widespread and available at virtually all major medical facilities, especially those specializing in cancer treatment. To the
contrary, it seems that palliative care teams are not widely available,
even at major medical facilities.*

*We believe that these misconceptions—by the general public, medi-
cal professionals, and healthcare administrators—poorly serve men
with prostate cancer at any stage and should be corrected.*

*Research has clearly shown that the delivery of palliative care to
men with prostate cancer at all stages of development has a positive
impact on those men and their families—both psychologically and
physiologically. That more men do not have access to palliative care
and its benefits during their treatment is tragic, and it is a situation that
must be corrected.*

17

Beyond Intimacy, Maintaining Perspective

While the development of prostate cancer will change much of your day-to-day world, it need not be the end of it. Yes, it is likely that your sexual capabilities will change, some dramatically. And your emotional perspective on and reaction to the world around you will change. But change can be a positive, too, and it can give you and your partner or spouse an opportunity to further develop the existing closeness of your relationship.

While such positive outcomes—besides "beating cancer"—can occur during your battle with the disease, it is not a given that you'll be successful. A key point often stated by professionals dealing with prostate cancer patients is that strong relationships can be strengthened by the challenges of this disease. Other relationships, where communications are already strained, may weaken even further or completely fall apart.

The one certain outcome of your battle with prostate cancer is that you and your partner will have an opportunity to test the integrity of your relationship, and, with a bit of luck, actually strengthen that relationship. A therapist can be a great help and should be engaged as early as possible in your treatment process.

When you are told that "you might have prostate cancer," your whole emotional and psychological worlds are changed, sometimes even upended. Regardless of whether you are married, have children (and, perhaps, grandchildren), are single, or in a relationship with an intimate or friendly partner, one thing is certain: *Your world will change.*

First, your very physiology changes because the prospect of having prostate cancer sets in motion an array of emotional stimuli and defense responses that alter the core chemistry of your body. How it functions—or doesn't function—will change, too.

All of these elements—your physical and emotional conditions, your interpersonal relationships, your vision of the future, your concept of mortality, and especially your self-image—constitute your emotional aura (which we discussed in detail earlier in this book.). They influence who you are, what you do, and how you view life and all its facets. They determine how you react to the words and emotions of those who surround you.

Because your emotional aura literally encompasses the whole of your being, it is critically important to understand how the many aspects of your being will change, and what you can do to control them, and thus how you react to the world around you.

Critical to this process are two factors:

1. Fully understanding your prostate cancer condition.
2. Securing a knowledgeable and compatible counselor to help you (and your partner) understand and gain perspective about your condition and the decisions you will have to make about your future.

Experts believe that obtaining a knowledgeable counselor is a vital element of prostate cancer treatment, yet it is one that is absent in many cases. Here are the sad facts of this medical shortcoming, according to a *Newsweek* magazine report in July 2017:

> At least 60% of cancer survivors suffer from long-term sexual problems, and fewer than 20 percent get the help they need to lead fulfilling sex lives, says Leslie Schover, a clinical psychologist who is one of the pioneers in helping cancer survivors navigate sexual health and fertility.
>
> Only half of all cancer patients recall anyone from oncology addressing the effects that treatment will have on sex and intimacy, and just 20% report being satisfied with the help they received from healthcare professionals for their sexual problems.[1]

Those numbers are devastating! And unfortunately, the lack of professional help provided to prostate cancer patients and their spouses is not uncommon and may result in tragedy. The following is one woman's story of woe and her plaintive search for understanding, as reported in MedHelp.[2]

It's been three-and-a-half years since my husband's prostate cancer surgery. We have not been able to have sex in that time. He's tried all the pills and injections, [but] nothing works. In this time, we have grown so far apart it's ridiculous. Been married for 30 years and I want to leave, that's all I can think about.

I want to have a physical relationship again. I didn't think it would be this bad when he was first diagnosed. But this is affecting me too much. I told him a year ago that I didn't want to be married anymore, but I stayed.

Now I feel that I need to make a move. I know he will be hurt, but I need to be happy again. I have never been so sad in my entire life. . . . I just need to be with someone that can make me happy again. Has anyone been through this before?

However, that same *Newsweek* article provides at least a glimmer of hope when the author states: "There are therapies and medications available to every patient, along with a small cadre of experts who help survivors navigate the jagged path back to sexual health—if only patients and doctors would learn how to talk about it."

But here, too, the situation is problematic. Attempting, much less achieving, sexual intimacy after cancer is "predicated on one assumption: Oncologists and patients talking about the ways cancer affects sexuality and interventions that can help." Most healthcare professionals, however, have little if any training on sexuality. And "healthcare providers, especially oncologists, are not trained how to ask about it. Sex is an issue that goes unmentioned."[3]

Reflecting on the tragic condition of the women cited above, the logical questions is: "What can I, as a partner, expect?" As we know by now, "One of the effects of prostate cancer treatment is erectile dysfunction or impotence. This means that a woman's male partner may not be able to have erections that are hard enough for him to have sex." The physiological and psychological conditions affect not only the man but also his partner. As UCLA Health cautions:[4]

If you are the partner of a man with erectile dysfunction, it can be difficult to cope with changes in your sexual relationship. Sometimes men struggle to come to terms with changes in their body image or their ability to perform sexually. This can sometimes result in him staying away from intimate situations where he may feel under pressure to make love.

UCLA Health advises that such a reaction is only natural, but that "you may feel rejected by what seems like a lack of sexual interest or intimacy. This may not have anything to do with his feelings for you but is a result of his cancer treatment. [Nonetheless] erectile dysfunction can be difficult for both of you."

So, what's next? How can you, as a partner, help him and help yourself, too. A good start, UCLA Health suggests, is to reassure your partner that:

- He is no less of a man to you, and that
  - Sex is not as important as long as he is healthy.
  - You will work through it with him.
  - That you understand his feelings.
- He remains important to you.
- Nonsexual touching and intimacy such as kissing and cuddling are important to you.

If, however, sex is very important to both of you, then this "may be an opportunity for you to experiment sexually with each other and work on ways to remain intimate, even when an erection is not possible." On the issue of finding to ways of being sexually satisfied, UCLA doctors further suggests the following:

There are many different ways to be sexual. Take this time to explore together the things you can do with each other that are sexually exciting. Explore a variety of options to maintain sexual and emotional intimacy and satisfaction.

If you are used to your partner being the sexual initiator, this may be the time for a little role-reversal. It is OK for you to tell your partner that even though he has erectile dysfunction, you want to stay in touch physically and intimately. Talk to your partner about ways to do this.

Instead of trying to 'fix your sex life' take this as a time to "play."

Finally, they also suggest, "don't hesitate to talk to your partner's doctor or healthcare team, if you are having difficulties with your partner's erectile dysfunction." Counseling is an educational process, and it should begin before the man begins treatment.

In addition to conditioning the patient and his partner about the outcomes that can be expected after surgery, counseling can enhance the effectiveness of erectile dysfunction medications and "help improve couples' sex lives," according to a study published online in *Cancer*, a peer-reviewed journal of the American Cancer Society. Furthermore, "both Internet-based counseling and face-to-face therapy sessions improved the sex lives of prostate cancer survivors and their spouses," according to an ABC News report, which cited the 2011 study led by Dr. Leslie Schover, then a psychologist and professor at the University of Texas MD Anderson Cancer Center in Houston.[5] (Dr. Schover retired from Houston's Anderson Center in 2016 and is now a leading force at Will2Love.com, an online counseling site to which she devotes herself full time. Will2Love.com seeks to optimize care for cancer-related problems with sex and fertility, including "online self-help tools for men and women, online training and support for oncology health professionals, and consulting to hospitals on how to structure a reproductive health program" according to the website.)

Reporting on Dr. Schover's study, HealthDay, an online healthcare information site, wrote that while the side effects of prostate cancer treatments can seriously disrupt a couple's sex life, her research showed, "Counseling helped married men and women figure out what sorts of treatments for erectile dysfunction worked for them and how to incorporate those methods during sex. In doing so, they returned some luster to their love lives."[6]

For the study, researchers enrolled more than 200 men who had been treated for prostate cancer and their wives into one of three groups to receive either:

- Face-to-face counseling
- Internet-based counseling
- Placement on a counseling wait list

At a six-month follow-up, the men who received either the face-to-face or internet-based counseling reported an improvement in sexual function and satisfaction with sex. The results showed a connection between a man's self-report (that the man's sexual functions had improved) with his wife's equally positive report. Those in the wait-listed group experienced no improvements, which suggested that "time alone doesn't heal the issues," according to Dr. Schover, who added, "Every subscale improved except desire, which we weren't surprised by because very few had low desire to begin with, so there wasn't that far to go on that."

According to the HealthDay report, men and women in the study were given questionnaires that asked about sexual function and sexual satisfaction, including their erectile function, the ability to achieve orgasm, and their level of desire. It reported that men's ability to achieve "near-normal" erections improved after counseling. Before counseling, about 12 percent to 15 percent of men reported few erection difficulties. That increased to between 36% and 44% for those who underwent counseling.

At the one-year mark, men reported that their sexual function and satisfaction results that were about the same as healthy men, according to Dr. Bruce Gilbert, director of reproductive and sexual medicine at the Smith Institute for Urology.[7] It is important to note that the results of the study were derived from a small sampling that spanned a short period of time and that 34 percent of couples enrolled dropped out for unknown reasons. Nonetheless, Dr. Gilbert noted, "A study like this is very important and highlights that there is a lot that happens if you engage couples or the patient in some type of counseling."

Couples and physicians should also never forget that while prostate cancer is frightening, so is the worry of patients that even if it is cured, "they may not be the same after a procedure than before," Gilbert said. "That's a real fear for men." Experts also suggest that if you're not getting all the help you need from your urologist, ask for a referral to a urologist who specializes in sexual medicine or a mental health professional.

IN OUR OPINION. . .

We believe that among the most important messages you can take from this book is an understanding that professional counselors—personal decision assistants, sex counselors, palliative care specialists, or others—can be critical to your successful recovery and your fight with and after prostate cancer.

Earlier in this book, we devoted a full chapter to the subject of professional counselors. Here, we have described but one aspect of your life's adaptation to prostate cancer—sex. That little-talked-about subject that is all but taboo in much of polite American conversation comes to the forefront when we deal with prostate cancer. We believe that if a successful recovery from prostate cancer treatment—and its aftermath—is going to be achieved, it will be more fully and quickly accomplished with the assistance of a professional prostate cancer counselor, not just any counselor.

Section 5

RECURRENT PROSTATE CANCER,
A BIOCHEMICAL RECURRENCE

18

What If My Prostate Cancer Returns?

Among the numerous ways to define prostate cancer is that it is "insidious." It is stealthy and treacherous, subtle and wily. It lurks in the background, slowly developing until you discover it, which, one hopes, is soon enough to tackle the demon and conquer it.

Such is the silent demonic nature that is recurrent prostate cancer.

The process seems recurrent. First you discovered it, treated it, hoped you killed the beast—but now you discover that it has slinked back and lurks once again. This is called a biochemical recurrence (BCR).

Fortunately, though, oncologists, research teams, and physicians are continually trying new drugs in clinical use and in experimental clinical trials, and both are having success. And the survival rate is increasing.

While that is the good news—that the survival rate is increasing—not all of the news is good.

If a man discovers his prostate cancer and is treated early, he may enjoy many cancer-free years. However, he should not overlook the fact that ZEROCancer.org says, "40% of men will experience a recurrence."[1] *American Journal of Managed Care* put it even higher, at between 20 percent and 50 percent.[2] Understandably, such a recurrence can be depressing and cause some men, and their families, to become disgusted with the whole taxing process of treating and attempting to manage their disease.

However, such naturally negative reactions need not be the case. Texas Oncology, a cancer treatment group, says that, "Recent advances in treatment have resulted in new . . . options that reduce symptoms and improve survival."[3]

Typically, the first sign of a recurrent prostate cancer is a rising prostate-specific antigen (PSA), which begins well before any clinical signs or symptoms of the disease. So, then, the first key questions are:

- At what level is a rising PSA to be of concern?
- Is the rate of the PSA's increase important?
- At what point should additional treatment be considered?
- Which treatments should be attempted?

It is important for men to understand that the PSA is a marker for prostate cancer activity, not just the progression of the disease. However, the PSA level is "an important way of understanding how your prostate cancer is progressing," writes the Prostate Cancer Foundation. (The PCF produced an excellent and understandable series of booklets about prostate cancer that are worth your attention.)

Men should remember that prostate-specific antigens, or PSAs, are produced by all prostate cells, not just prostate cancer cells. However, while your cancer cells have either been removed through surgery, effectively killed by radiation, or deprived of life-giving serums through chemicals such as ADT, some cells may still have spread outside the treatment areas before they could be removed or killed. Or the treatment could have missed a few of the cancer cells. "These [escaped] cells at some point begin to multiply and produce enough PSA that it can again become detectable" by lab tests, says the PCF.

Treating recurring cancer is broadly determined by two variables:

1. The extent of your cancer
2. The treatment you previously received

Three indicators of recurrent prostate cancer are:

1. An increase in your PSA reading
2. Evidence in X-rays
3. Evidence in bone scans

Follow-up treatment is based on whether your earlier treatment was surgery, radiation, hormone therapy, or a combination of some or all three.

RECURRENT PROSTATE CANCER AFTER SURGERY

That some elements of the prostate cancer remain in your system is not uncommon, especially in the case of surgical removal of the prostate, called a prostatectomy. Dr. Marc B. Garnick, a Harvard prostate cancer expert, says if your PSA begins to rise after treatment, four key questions will help determine your next steps:

1. What were your risk characteristics, such as Gleason score, PSA, and cancer stage at the time of diagnosis?
2. What type of treatment(s) did you have?
3. How long has it been since you underwent initial therapy for prostate cancer? This will help indicate how aggressive follow-up treatment needs to be.
4. How fast is your PSA rising?

Your oncology team may recommend either watchful waiting or further treatment. The follow-up treatment selection will be based on where the team believes the cancer is located and will be preceded by treatment tests such as CTs, MRIs, or bone scans to define the location(s) as accurately as possible. If the cancer is thought to be in your prostate area, a second surgical procedure might be recommended.

If it has spread outside the prostate, the most likely destinations are your nearby lymph nodes, and then your bones, lungs, liver, brain, or other organs. In that case, the American Cancer Society (ACS) believes that "hormone therapy is probably the most effective treatment. But it isn't likely to cure the cancer, and at some point, it might stop working."[4] "If you've had a radical prostatectomy, radiation therapy might be an option, sometimes along with hormone therapy," according to the American Cancer Society. If you've already had radiation therapy, however, having additional radiation therapy is not usually an option because of the increased risk of serious side effects. Once you have received radiation therapy directed toward the prostate gland, "more radiation therapy typically cannot be given to the same area safely."[5] Your next option could be cryotherapy or radical prostatectomy. However, these treatments carry higher risks of side effects such as incontinence, especially when performed after radiation treatment.

In the case of brachytherapy (seed implantation), however, radiation may be an option. If the location of the cancer is not clear and the only indication is an elevated PSA level, then active surveillance, or watchful waiting, may be the recommendation. Since prostate cancer is often slow growing, it might not cause problems for years. A Johns Hopkins University study of men whose PSA levels began to rise after surgery, for example, found that, on average, it was about ten years before the cancer showed signs of having spread to other parts of a man's body.

A key question about recurrent prostate cancer after prostate surgery is whether it has metastasized (spread) to other part of the body. If it has not spread and is localized to the area of the prostate, then radiation therapy may be used, along with Androgen Deprivation Therapy (ADT) or other chemotherapy. Chemotherapy is used to treat recurrent prostate cancer in areas distant from the prostate because of its ability to improve survival.[6]

If your recurrent cancer has spread to other parts of your body, then ADT is often the primary method of treating it. "Systemic treatment with ADT is the mainstay of treatments for individuals with recurrent prostate cancer following primary treatment with radiation," Texas Oncology reports. Surgical removal of the prostate following radiation treatment is rare, and cryosurgery is ineffective at this stage. Therefore, chemotherapy or immunotherapy are the procedures typically used.

The purpose of ADT is to reduce the level of male hormones, such as testosterone, which "feed" the prostate cancer cells—or to prevent them from entering cells and influencing their behavior. ADT treatment for prostate cancer patients may control growth of the cancer for a few years; "However, most prostate cancers stop responding to this treatment and begin to grow again. Cancers that grow in spite of ADT are called hormone-refractory (HRPC)," Texas Oncology further explains. In such cases, treatments may include chemotherapy, immunotherapy, additional hormonal therapy or participation in clinical studies that are evaluating new treatments. Occasionally, local radiation therapy may be used to alleviate symptoms of the cancer.

It is important to note that the drugs, treatments, and therapies we write about in this and other sections are not exhaustive lists. Oncology teams are continuously developing, testing, and conducting clinical trials on potential new solutions.

NEW CANCER THERAPIES AND HOW THEY WORK

Chemotherapy

Chemotherapy is systemic in that the cancer-fighting drugs injected into the body will circulate and reach locations where the cancer has spread; this process attempts to kill or eliminate the cancers cells.

Several chemotherapeutic drugs may be used in this effort, including mitoxantrone (Novantrone®), docetaxel (Taxotere®), paclitaxel, and Estramustine.® Texas Oncology reports that all "have some effectiveness in treating prostate cancer."

Hormone Therapy

Hormonal medications have been developed and approved by the FDA to inhibit the synthesis of androgen and block androgen receptors. They are now used to treat metastatic prostate cancer following chemotherapy treatment.[7, 8]

Abiraterone Zytiga®—Abiraterone blocks the production of androgens in the testes and in the adrenal glands as well as the tumor itself. When administered with prednisone, Abiraterone has resulted in improved quality of life and delayed HRPC patients' reports of pain progression.

Although Abiraterone is "generally well-tolerated, side effects may include fatigue, high blood pressure and electrolyte or liver abnormalities and patients need to be monitored regularly," Texas Oncology research finds.[9]

Enzalutamide Xtandi®—Enzalutamide targets multiple steps in the androgen-receptor–signaling pathway, interfering with molecular pathways that help the prostate cancer grow. Of considerable personal importance for patients, the drug does not cause the side effects commonly associated with chemotherapy, such as nausea and hair loss. Enzalutamide has been shown to improve survival, reduce the risk of cancer progression, and delay the need for additional chemotherapy in men with HRPC," according to Texas Oncology.

Immunotherapy

Biological therapy is a treatment that uses the body's immune system to help kill cancer cells. It also may be referred to as immunologic therapy, immunotherapy, or biotherapy. Biologic therapies developed for the treatment of prostate cancer include interferon, interleukin, monoclonal antibodies, colony stimulating factors (cytokines) and vaccines.

Men with advanced metastatic prostate cancer that is resistant to hormone therapy are candidates for Sipuleucel-T (PROVENGE®), which prompts the body's immune system to respond against the cancer. Because of the response it causes, PROVENGE is considered an immunotherapy, according to Dana-Farber/Brigham & Women's Cancer Institute (DF/BWCI).

"The vaccine is produced by removing some of a patient's white blood cells, then exposing them to a protein from prostate cancer cells and a stimulatory molecule," DF/BWCI explains on its website. "This process primes the white cells to attack prostate cancer when they are re-injected into the body."

To evaluate the effect of Sipuleucel-T (PROVENGE), the first treatment of its type to be FDA approved for men with metastatic, androgen-independent prostate cancer, researchers conducted a phase III clinical trial known as IMPACT, or Immunotherapy for Prostate Adenocarcinoma Treatment.[10] That trial enrolled 512 men who were treated with either Sipuleucel-T or a placebo and then directly compared. Results of the trial show that:

Median survival time was

- 25.8 months among men treated with PROVENGE versus 21.7 months among men treated with placebo.

Three-year survival was

- 31.7 percent among men treated with Sipuleucel-T versus 23 percent among men treated with placebo.
- Sipuleucel-T did not significantly delay cancer progression.[11, 12]

The side effects associated with use of Sipuleucel-T included chills, fever, and headaches, most of which were low grade and of short duration.

Novel Immunotherapies

Novel immunotherapies are vaccine strategies that harness the immune system and include such substances as PROSTVAC and Ipilimumab, which is a monoclonal anti-CTLA4 antibody that binds to a receptor on T cells, blocking CTLA4.

Other vaccines are in the works. One is called PROSTVAC-VF (also called PSA-TRICOM) that uses a modified smallpox virus as its means of entry into the body and targets any cell that makes PSA. PROSTVAC is being tested in a worldwide clinical trial called the Prospect Trial, which involves 1,200 men with metastatic CRPC (castration resistant prostate cancer) from about 200 centers. If the trial results investigators are waiting for show positive performance as well as they expect, then men could start getting this vaccine in addition to PROVENGE.[13]

Another vaccine, GVAX, is being tested by Dr. Charles G. Drake of the Johns Hopkins Kimmel Cancer Center and geneticist Dr. Stylianos E. Antonarakis, also associated with Johns Hopkins. The test is among men with high-risk prostate cancer who are undergoing surgery. The trials are to determine if the immune system can be activated to attack the cancer.

BONE COMPLICATIONS

Among patients with advanced prostate cancer, the disease has spread, or metastasized, to their bones. Bone metastases often cause these effects:

- Pain
- An increase the risk of fractures
- A possible increase in the amount of calcium in the blood (hypercalcemia), which is a life-threatening condition

Treatments for bone complications may include radiation or drug therapy, such as the following:

- "Zoledronic acid (Zometa®) may be used to reduce the risk of complications (bone loss) from bone metastases or to treat cancer-related hypercalcemia," according to Texas Oncology. The loss of bone occurs when the cancer has spread, which increases the risk of fractures and pain.
- Denosumab (Xgeva™) targets a protein known as the RANK ligand, which regulates cells that break down the bone. "Deno-sumab was better than zoledronic acid for prevention of skeletal-related events, and potentially represents a novel treatment option in men with bone metastases from castration-resistant prostate cancer."[14]
- Xofigo® Radium Ra 223 dichloride is a targeted radio-pharmaceutical agent that binds with minerals in the bone to deliver radiation directly to bone tumors. This delivery method limits damage to normal surrounding tissues. Texas Oncology states that "pain from bone metastases may also be relieved with radiation therapy directed to the affected bones."
- Custirsen inhibits your body's production of custirsen, which is a protein associated with treatment resistance in prostate cancer as well as in other cancers.
- Orteronel is an inhibitor that is currently being tested in a phase III trial comparing Orteronel and prednisone to placebo and prednisone.
- Tiquinamide is an "orally active drug that has antiangiogenic (pre-vents blood vessel growth in the cancer) activity and other anticancer properties. It is currently in ongoing phase III clinical trials," according to Texas Oncology.

IN OUR OPINION. . .

The one truism about prostate cancer is that, broadly stated, the later in life that you discover its onset, the better. While this rationale may seem a bit morbid, it is realistic. This is because if your doctor catches the existence of prostate cancer in its early stages and you are older—thus, with less life to live—the greater are your chances of dying with the disease than dying of the disease.

Since nearly all men with low- to intermediate-grade prostate cancer (the most common types) can expect to live at least five years after the initial diagnosis, men who are in their eighties are likely to fulfill that cliché, since the average life expectancy for American men is in the range of eighty to eighty-five. Likewise, on average, 98 percent of men will survive ten years past the detection of their prostate cancer, and 95 percent will survive fifteen years. "Since many men who get prostate cancer are already elderly, they are more likely to die from causes other than the cancer," says WebMD.

At the outset, you may not find those statistics particularly reassuring, but if you think about the scenario, they are actually positive numerical outcomes, and those outcomes give you much better mortality odds than if you were a younger man. Thus, there's at least some advantage of being an older man.

If you are fifty when the cancer is discovered, however, then your prospects are not so good; you have an increased chance of dying of *prostate cancer,* not *with it.*

Regardless of age, however, oncology researchers continue to develop new drugs and conduct numerous clinical trials in their efforts to forestall the inevitable.

Section 6

LOOKING TOWARD THE FUTURE

19

What Does the Future Hold for Me?

One of the most amazing human traits is our ability to adapt to change—to new, different, and sometimes troublesome conditions and challenges. This ability is a fortunate aspect of our human makeup because dealing with prostate cancer and its treatments require you to change, to adapt, and to accommodate the many alterations that will take place in both your body and mind.

To successfully manage the physiological changes, you must first achieve a positive psychological outlook.

A typical outcome—of changes in your body and its behavior—is depression, which can accommodate urinary incontinence, fecal incontinence, and erectile dysfunction, among others. These are all realities of prostate cancer treatments and likely were noted—if only in passing—by your oncology team. Whether you internalized and seriously considered the impact of these predictions, however—and whether you actually realized the impact they would have on your life—is something quite different.

This chapter deals more with the mental and philosophical aspects of the impact of treatment. The following chapter, "How Long Will My Recovery Take?" deals with more specific recovery challenges.

Your doctor looks at your lab results, X-rays, scans, sheaves of papers, scrolls down a computer screen, and responds to what he sees: "All good." You have survived your treatments well, your overall health is good, and best of all, and your PSA is low, so "all good."

Yes, your oncologist is satisfied with the empirical examination of your body, and he considers his work a success and nearly complete—although there will be years of follow-up exams, probably until you die.

And so, it may be "all good" from his perspective because his big job is largely over. However, your journey continues, and in more than a few cases, your trek will be a challenging one. Yes, your reports are "all good," but one big question remains, "What shape are you really in?"

Oncologists are trained in medicine and the very-detailed specifics of cancer, but this training likely has not stressed the physical and psychological challenges that you will face as a prostate cancer survivor. That's because those facets of the disease don't really "connect" with a doctor's training.

Naturally, therefore, your doctor is somewhat detached from the not-so-subtle psychological and emotional aspects of your recovery. While your doctor can sympathize with your plight, dealing with your personal problems and your personal recovery challenges must be faced and hopefully surmounted by you.

Unfortunately, there seems to be little, if any, thought given by medical teams to what level of support or guidance you will need after your oncology treatment is completed, or what counseling you should receive to successfully reenter "normal" life. In fact, formal counseling, guidance, and support programs for post–prostate cancer treatment patients may not even exist in your community.

While the medical treatment may be finite and now largely accomplished, your challenges will endure for the rest of your life, and they can significantly impact your quality of life.

Fortunately, patient-centered, high-value "psychosocial care has been shown to improve patient outcomes and survival, offset medical costs, and reduce unnecessary emergency room use," wrote Dr. Ellen Miller-Sonet in the May 10, 2019, newsletter of the American Society of Clinical Oncologists.[1]

While your hospital may provide only limited psychosocial support for prostate and other cancer survivors, at least three national groups do more.

- Us TOO is an international organization that provides "educational resources, support services and personal connections to the prostate cancer community."[2] The organization's goals are to "transform resignation into determination and fear into hope." It seeks these goals through in-person and online services newsletters, educational materials, and events.

  With more than 200 support chapters worldwide, Us TOO actively involves itself in the recovery process of prostate cancer patients. Although global in scope, its headquarters is in Des Plaines, Illinois, and the website is USTOO.com. It can be contacted at 800-808-7866.

- CancerCare.org was founded in 1944 in New York City as a nonprofit 501(c)(3) group that deals with cancer patients broadly, not just prostate cancer patients.

"CancerCare is committed to helping people affected by cancer cope with psychosocial issues by providing high-quality emotional and social support. Through our comprehensive network of support services, anyone anywhere can get help," according to the organization's press materials.

The organization provides counseling, support groups, workshops, publications, community programs, and financial and co-pay assistance. CancerCare.org is "a leading national, nonprofit organization [that] helps people cope with and manage both the emotional and practical challenges of cancer. All of our services are provided by professional oncology social workers dedicated to supporting people affected by cancer." To learn more, call 800-813-HOPE (4673) or visit www.cancercare.org/services org.

- Cancer Support Community is a nonprofit 502(c)(3), and its motto is "No one faces cancer alone." With headquarters in Washington, DC, the organization has major biopharma companies as its partners and founders.

In March 2019, the CSC established a "strategic partnership" with Airbnb that "will provide free housing for cancer patients and caregivers, if they meet certain geographic and income criteria."

The organization provides information and support for individuals living with cancer, information on how friends and family can "make a difference," and research and policy advocacy outreach. They operate 9 a.m. to 9 p.m., Monday through Friday, and their hotline number is 888-793-9355.

Additionally, many hospitals that specialize in treating the many phases of prostate cancer have "support groups" that may provide help for you in enduring the process. One way to find your local prostate cancer support group is for you or your spouse to ask your doctor how you might contact one. Or use your computer and search for "prostate cancer support group" *and* your local city or hospital name. Following are some results from a Google search.

- Prostate Cancer Foundation, https://www.pcf.org/patient-resources/patient-navigation/support-groups/
- Cancer Support Community, https://www.cancersupportcommunity.org/prostate-cancer
- CancerCare, https://www.cancercare.org/support_groups/126-prostate_cancer_patient_support_group
- Prostate Cancer Research Institute, https://pcri.org/supportgroups
- National Alliance of State Prostate Cancer Coalitions, https://naspcc.org/index.php/resources/prostate-cancer-patient-online-support-group
- American Cancer Society, https://www.cancer.org/treatment/support-programs-and-services.html

IN OUR OPINION. . .

As you know very well by now, there few certainties in life, and even fewer with prostate cancer. About the only thing we know for certain is that if your prostate cancer metastasizes and if you do not die from another cause, you will die of prostate cancer. While that is not a very pleasant thought, it is one of the few certainties we have in life.

With that morbid thought behind us, let's next examine why this is the case: most doctors are highly specialized and very knowledgeable about a specific area of detection and treatment. They often treat a specific disease or collection of similar diseases.

While a cancer treatment hospital may suggest that it has an integrated plan of working with patients afflicted with dramatic and sometimes fatal diseases like prostate cancer, the reality is that few facilities employ a fully unified approach to treating both a disease and the patient. Although several organizations provide psychological support and assistance in treating the disease, it is uncommon for a single institution to address all of a patient's unique blend of needs—physiological, psychological, palliative, religious, and rehabilitative, among others.

20

How Long Will My Recovery Take?

Cancer doesn't have an on/off switch. Rather, cancer is a continuous journey. Even after your treatment ends, it is probable that you will find life is not the same as it was before. The cancer, its various treatments, or simply the passage of time will have taken their toll.

Not being able to return to "normal" can be frustrating. Those words seek to provide some comfort in a time of anxiety, physical change, and even thoughts of suicide. Indeed, those words fall far short in facing the challenges that lie ahead.

Let's be bluntly honest about this: your body and your life have changed. They will never be as they were before prostate cancer treatment. You will face significant physical and emotional challenges; you can use all the intelligent and caring help you can get from your family (and professionals) who understand the ravages prostate cancer has wrought on your body and mind—and that likely will continue.

Prostate cancer is no game, and it will forever leave you with scars—both physical and psychological. So, the advice of ZERO Cancer is worth your attention. They say that "Life after treatment . . . may be scary and destabilizing to you, but it's important not to be intimidated by the path ahead. Take the time you need to recover and consider the following tips:

- Don't expect to recover instantly (and don't expect to recover completely).
- Receive (graciously) the understanding of your family and community.

- Develop new hobbies or interests to fit with your abilities and limitations.

Now, let's deal with the specific conditions and changes you may have to deal with during life following prostate cancer.

FATIGUE

"Cancer-related fatigue is one of the most common side effects of cancer and its treatment. It usually comes on suddenly, is not a result of activity or exertion, and is not relieved by rest or sleep."[1] So writes the Cleveland Clinic on its website. Cancer cells are competing with and depriving normal growth cells of nutrients. Decreased nutrition may result from nausea, vomiting, mouth sores, taste changes, heartburn, or diarrhea. Side effects of some medicines cause nausea, pain, depression, and anxiety, all of which cause fatigue. Finally, the clinic says, "Depression and fatigue often go hand-in-hand, [and] it may not be clear which started first."[2] Fatigue has several possible causes:

- Lower blood count, especially caused by chemotherapy can lead to anemia
- Stress, as well as chronic severe pain, increases fatigue
- Overtaxing your body by trying to maintain your traditional daily routine may cause fatigue

While many authorities agree that fatigue will decrease over time, coping with it for an extended period of time may be necessary. ZERO Cancer suggests seven ways to deal with fatigue after prostate surgery.[3]

- Eat a nutritious diet (discussed later in this book).
- Set realistic goals for your daily accomplishments.
- Schedule your high-effort activities for the times when you have the most energy.
- Get eight hours of sleep nightly.
- Rest during each day.
- Be physically active, but only to a comfortable level.
- Allow others to help you and ask for their assistance.

DEPRESSION

Dealing with prostate cancer–related depression is essential, not just for the man who continues to deal with the disease and its aftermath but also for those close to him. The Prostate Cancer Foundation (PCF) notes that while the recovery process can be tough on men as they try to return to their normal lives, "Only recently has the effect on wives and family been addressed."

A study by the European Association of Urology (EAU) revealed that "Many wives of advanced prostate cancer sufferers feel that their lives are being undermined by their husband's illness, with nearly half reporting that their own health suffered," the PCF reported. It says, somewhat prosaically, that, "No matter why you have depression, don't worry. You are not alone." Their suggestions are similarly banal:

- Seek medical attention for changes in attitude.
- Find and join a support group.
- Talk to family and friends.
- Write expressively—writing about your experience can lessen the mental effects.

"Depression is a mood disorder in which persistent feelings of sadness interfere with (your) ability to participate in normal activities," according to ZERO Cancer: 'This feeling of depression can manifest itself in a sense of vulnerability, sadness, a fear of recurrent prostate cancer or even death. These can lead to more disability problems with intense anxiety or panic."

While some advice about dealing with depression after prostate cancer treatment simply suggests talking with your "medical team," not everyone has access to such a "team" to talk with. Two organizations, CancerCare and Us TOO International, surveyed 633 patients with prostate cancer regarding their feelings of anxiety and depression" and revealed the following stark results.[4]

- 77 percent of the respondents said they had symptoms of anxiety or depression following their prostate cancer diagnosis.
- 94 percent of the respondents thought it was normal for patients with prostate cancer to feel anxiety and depression.

- 97 percent of the respondents believed there was a need to help patients recognize these symptoms and find treatment for them.

Those results represent virtual unanimity and emphasizes the urgent need to address depression and anxiety among prostate cancer patients. Professional prostate cancer teams need to pay attention. Sadly, and as we have noted earlier in this book, *Oncology Nursing News* (*ONN*) reported that:

> Men tend not to seek out help for psycho-social issues—notably less often than women do. This is borne out by survey results that suggest men with prostate cancer would benefit from support groups, yet they seldom attend them, and other data shows that women outnumber men by three-to-one in cancer support groups.

The publication suggested that, "There are often feelings of embarrassment and shame attached to their diagnosis" of prostate cancer because of "adverse events such as incontinence and erectile dysfunction." As a result, "these factors may lead the patient to hide his feelings even more deeply from medical staff and to refrain from divulging his feelings to his family and loved ones." *ONN* notes that clinicians should be aware that "Men diagnosed with prostate cancer may already feel diminished in the eyes of others and, subsequently, may reject the interventions that can help mitigate anxiety and depression." It adds that support groups, counseling, and antianxiety or antidepressant medications, which may all be highly useful, are seen as "further signs of weakness."

While *ONN* agrees with the PCF on the need to deal with these problems, *ONN* nevertheless takes a stand and stresses that clinical teams should "make clear that these interventions are often helpful and may lead to a better quality of life and improved medical outcomes."

While we have accurately summarized here Andrew Chesler's study in *ONN*, it would be worth your time to read the full piece.[5]

LASTING CHANGES

While the changes to your body from prostate cancer treatment are euphemistically called "side effects," many are actually enduring and will impact the core of your being for the rest of your life. These include, but are not limited to, the following:

- Erectile dysfunction, impotence
- Urinary incontinence
- Fecal incontinence

While some doctors utter wishful predictions and tell you that you will return to "normal" in several months, the truth of the matter is that a genuine "return to normal" seldom happens. And, if it does, it will be for a very small percentage of men who have undergone prostate cancer treatment: the "new normal" of your post-treatment world will be quite different from the "normal" you have been accustomed to. Recovery from and accommodating to the changes in your body will begin the moment you awaken from surgery—or following hormone or radiation treatment—and they will be lifelong.

Erectile Dysfunction

While the effects of prostate cancer treatment vary from man to man, erectile dysfunction (ED, or impotence) is a "very common side effect [among the] unwanted changes that may occur in your body during or after prostate cancer treatment," as UCLA Health describes it.[6] The university explains that ED is when "a man's penis cannot get hard enough for him to have sex," which clearly creates problems for a man and his sex partner. ED also eliminates a man's ability to masturbate.

Why does this happen? When a man is aroused, his brain instructs the nerves to his penis blood vessels to widen. When they do, blood flows into the penis—and outflow is decreased—causing it to harden. Unfortunately, all prostate treatments (surgery, radiation, and hormone) can or are likely to have negative effects on a man's bodily functions such as sexual arousal. The process of removing the prostate gland may damage or actually remove some of the nerves, blood vessels, and muscles employed by your body to create an erection, as well as to control your urination process. When this happens, your body ceases to function properly, such as allowing it to create an erection or controlling the sphincter function that regulates the flow of urine out of the bladder. "Your ability to have an erection after your surgery will depend on whether your prostate cancer was close to the nerves that control your erections, whether you had erections before surgery, as well as your age," according to UCLA Health.[7]

If you are able to have an erection after surgery, there will be no semen ejaculated when you have an orgasm, since semen is made by the prostate that was removed. While only 13 percent to 33 percent of the fluid in semen is produced by the prostate gland, it is a vital part of the reproductive process.[8]

There are two other main treatment-related causes of ED besides surgery:

- ED from radiation therapy—Like surgery, radiation therapy may damage the nerves in and near your prostate with the same negative impact on your sexual function. The doctors at Harvard Medical School state that from 30 to 70 percent of men treated with radiation will get ED, and 30 to 50 percent treated with brachytherapy will get ED. The onset of this dysfunction becomes more severe over six months or more following the completion of radiation therapy. In the absence of an erection, orgasm and ejaculation are not possible. This condition is permanent.
- ED from hormone therapy—Hormone therapy reduces the amount of testosterone in your body, but testosterone is the hormone that stimulates your interest in and ability to engage in sex. Hormone therapy may also result in erectile dysfunction—or you may maintain the desire to have sex but be unable to develop an erection or reach an orgasm. UCLA Health offers the hopeful note that, "Your ability to have an erection and your interest in sex may get better several months after your hormone treatment ends."

Urinary Incontinence

While incontinence can be associated with untreated prostate cancer, it is more often a side effect of prostate cancer treatments, according to the Mayo Clinic. Indeed, urinary incontinence is one of the most commonly reported side effects of radical prostatectomy for prostate cancer.

*Web*MD agrees that urinary incontinence is a commonplace consequence of prostate cancer surgery, including freezing (cryotherapy), radiation, and seed treatment (brachytherapy). Additionally, incontinence can result from an enlarged prostate known as benign prostatic hyperplasia (BPH).[9]

Estimates of the percentages of men who develop incontinence following a radical prostatectomy vary. Harvard estimates from 2 percent to 15 percent of patients "may develop incontinence."[10] The Cleveland Clinic estimates about half of that number: "Approximately 6% to 8% of men who have had surgery to remove their prostate will develop urinary incontinence."[11] Harvard suggests that the chances of developing incontinence after prostate surgery is

- 2 percent with eternal beam radiation.
- 1 percent to 2 percent with brachytherapy.

The development of urinary incontinence can occur along with the inability to achieve an erection. This becomes particularly problematic when these developments materialize after taking medications to stimulate an erection, thus making sexual intercourse technically possible. The irony is while your supplement (like Coverlet, discussed later) helps you develop an erection, your incontinence can release urine during attempted intercourse, which may make the event unpleasant for one or both parties. You might consider this a cruel twist of nature. "Incontinence and impotence are the evil twins of prostate cancer and its aftermath," wrote Dana Jennings in the *New York Times*:[12]

> While impotence can breed deep melancholy, incontinence is a more primal problem: Only babies and toddlers are supposed to wet themselves. Beyond those ages, it becomes a hushed subject, an object of shame, frustration, and bad jokes.

Whether incontinence is "a hushed subject" or not, it is a fact and an important problem that a significant number of men must face and manage in the aftermath of cancer treatment.

MedicineNet reports that "more than half of men in their 60s and up to 90% in their 70s and 80s" have some form of leakage or lower urinary tract symptoms, or LUTS. So, if you develop bladder problems, you are not unique. In fact, there are different types of urinary incontinence in men, which include stress incontinence, urge incontinence, and overflow incontinence. "Some men may have one, two, or all three types of incontinence," according to Dr. Melissa Conrad Stöppler in

MedicineNet.[13] She writes that "Treatment of urinary incontinence in men may include behavioral treatments, like bladder training (such as Kegel), exercises, medication, surgery or a combination of these therapies." While these treatments may provide little relief for men today, Dr. Stöppler notes that "Research is ongoing to discover new and better treatments for urinary incontinence in men."

We believe that while urinary incontinence may be written about somewhat casually—"Oh, yeh, urinary incontinence is when you gotta go a lot"—it is clearly not a matter of little consequence. The need for frequent urination can be quite limiting to your freedom of movement; for instance, you cannot be stuck on a plane or in a car unable to move for hours at a time. And it also is not uncommon for a man to suffer both urinary incontinences and nocturia, which causes a man to awaken frequently during the night to empty his bladder.

Table 20.1. Incidence of Prostate Cancer by Ethnic Groups

Incidence rates of new prostate cancer cases among five global socio-ethnic groups		Researchers note that cancer incidence and death rates vary among racial and ethnic groups, with rates generally highest among blacks and lowest among Asian-Pacific Islanders. Importantly, there are considerable differences within each of the broadly defined population groups described, despite scant data.
Black, non-Hispanic	198.4	
White, non-Hispanic	114.8	
Hispanic	104.9	
Native American	85.1	
Asian-Pacific Islander	63.5	
All races combined	123.2	

Source: Rebecca L. Siegel and Kimberly D. Miller, "Cancer Statistics, 2017," CA: *Cancer Journal for Clinicians*, January 5, 2017, https://onlinelibrary.wiley.com/doi/full/10.3322/caac.21387.

Urinary Incontinence Treatment

One Boston urologist says the problem of frequent urination is relatively common among all men over sixty, and that's especially the case by the time they reach their mid-seventies. But, he noted, men who have undergone radiation therapy for prostate cancer are almost assuredly candidates for frequent urination. Kegel pelvic exercises—scoffed at by some urologists—may provide some relief.

Voiding the bladder by limiting fluids to certain times of the day, for example, by reducing the intake of fluids in the afternoon, say by

4 p.m., or planning regular bathroom trips may also help control incontinence. The objective of this timed voiding or bladder training is to help you gain control and extend the time between trips to a bathroom.

Bladder training also includes Kegel exercises, which strengthen pelvic muscles that help hold urine in the bladder. The first step is to find the right muscles. Imagine that you are trying to stop yourself from passing gas. Squeeze the muscles you would use. If you sense a "pulling" feeling, those are the right muscles for pelvic exercises. Kegel exercises emphasize squeezing only pelvic muscles, not stomach or buttock muscles, which "can put more pressure on your bladder control muscles," according to MedicineNet. Your urologist likely can provide you with an instruction flyer on the Kegel procedures, which should be repeated several times a day with results beginning to appear in three to six weeks.

While the efficacy of Kegel is still debated, it is worth a try to help slow your frequent urination. *Web*MD suggests this: "Try squeezing your pelvic floor muscles for 3 seconds, then release for 3 seconds. Do this 10 times in a row."[14] They suggest working up to one set of ten Kegels two to three times a day. "Kegels aren't harmful," *Web*MD says. "In fact, you can make them a part of your daily routine. Do them while you're brushing your teeth, driving to work, eating dinner, or watching TV."

Despite a lack of scientific evidence that Kegel exercises work, one truism may well apply here: "The muscle you don't use is the muscle you lose." If frequent urination becomes a problem and is associated with the development of incontinence, however, Kegel may not work.

From experience, we believe that Kegel exercises are at least worth a try. For others, however, medicines (such as Ditropan XL or its generic version, Oxybutynin) may have value. (A very small number of men seek surgical assistance, discussed next in more detail.)

At present, most men with incontinence use absorbent pads or undergarments, which do little or nothing in dealing with the underlying causes but do address the impact of incontinence on a man's daily life—and his self-confidence about being in public.

For one of us, urinary incontinence did not become a problem until fifteen years after treatment, which consisted of a combination of surgery, radiation, and hormone therapies. It began as a small amount of leakage, then developed into regular and only slightly controlled leakage throughout the day *and* night. In between the leakage, I had to deal with frequent trips to the bathroom—and to quickly assess the availability of restrooms when in public. The frequency problem did not lessen at night and regular trips to the bathroom were commonplace.

Urinary and certainly fecal incontinence are no small issues, and it seems that medical science has had little success in devising a solution to these problems. We're waiting, doctors!

Medicines

Clearly, this is not a situation where "one size fits all" because, as MedicineNet notes, "some medicines can affect bladder control in different ways." They cite three specific examples of how medicine can treat incontinence.

- "Blocking abnormal nerve signals that make the bladder contract at the wrong time."
- Slowing the production of urine.
- Relaxing the bladder or shrinking the prostate (which in all likelihood does not apply to most men following prostate cancer treatment).

An example of this is a class of drugs called diuretics, which are often used to treat high blood pressure. They achieve this goal by reducing fluid in the body, but that increases urine production, which can result in the development of incontinence.

Therefore, if it is possible, some men may find that switching from a diuretic to another kind of blood pressure medicine takes care of their incontinence.[15] Such a switch of medications may be difficult, however, and will be unique in each situation.

Surgical Treatments

Another means of dealing with urinary incontinence is the artificial urinary sphincter, or AUS, according to Cleveland Clinic cancer specialists. "An artificial urinary sphincter can help patients who have moderate to severe urinary incontinence because they have had significant sphincter muscle or valve damage after prostate cancer surgery," according to the specialists. When the prostate cancer patient needs to urinate, he presses on a pump that controls the opening and closing of a cuff, which has been surgically placed around his upper urethra. This opens the cuff and allows urination. According to the Cleveland Clinic, the AUS procedure is successful in 90 percent of cases.

Other solutions to urinary incontinence include a urinary sling and urinary diversion. In the sling procedure, the surgeon creates an internal sling that keeps pressure on the urethra so that it does not open until the patient consciously releases the urine. The "urethral sling procedure is best suited for men who have mild to moderate urinary incontinence after a radical prostatectomy," and who remain unimproved by more conservative measures. "It is highly successful in helping patients overcome incontinence, or reduce episodes of leaking urine," according to the Cleveland Clinic.[16]

Yet another method of dealing with incontinence is "the urinary diversion solution." In this method of control, a surgeon first creates a reservoir and then an opening in the lower abdomen where the urine can be drained through a catheter into a bag.

Thus, while none of these solutions are particularly pleasant compared to normal urinary elimination, you can take some solace in the fact that there is a variety of possible solutions to your urinary incontinence problems.

Fecal Incontinence

In addition to urinary incontinence, fecal incontinence is not uncommon and is defined as "the inability to control the passage of stool—liquid or solid—or control flatus [gas]," according to MedicineNet.[17] Both urinary and fecal incontinence can result from damage to nerves, which is often the result of surgery or radiation therapy.

As stated earlier in this book—and perhaps not surprising—Dana-Farber's Dr. Sharon Bober says that, "some men find incontinence more difficult to deal with than impotence." That revelation, however, renders some men incredulous until they experience it firsthand. This raises the question: Which is worse? Having something you don't want, incontinence, or not having something that you do want, sexual potency?

A chief cause of fecal incontinence is external beam radiotherapy: it blankets a wide area with radiation, and with this treatment, the "bowel function tends to remain the same or deteriorate"—as the effects of radiation develop—rather than improve over time, according to the Prostate Cancer Foundation (PCF). Bowel dysfunction—including fecal incontinence as well as diarrhea and frequent stools—is more common following external beam radiotherapy than any other primary prostate cancer therapy, according to the PCF.

(During prostatectomy, damage to the anal-rectal area is about 2 percent to 3 percent. Following brachytherapy (seeds), bowel dysfunction tends to be lower than with external beam radiotherapy and seems to stabilize at a rate of less than 10 percent after one year.)

As the effects of radiation develop, "bowel function tends to remain the same or deteriorate rather than improve over time," according to Johns Hopkins. "After two years, about 10 percent to 20 percent of men reported having persistent diarrhea a few times each week, while rectal bleeding increased steadily from 5 percent immediately after treatment to 25 percent after two years."[18]

"By contrast, with brachytherapy, the rates of bowel dysfunction associated with intensity-modulated radiation therapy (IMRT) remain low after two years, hovering around 5 percent," Johns Hopkins continued, "Bowel dysfunction following brachytherapy tends to be lower than that seen with external beam radiotherapy, and, most importantly, seems to stabilize at a low rate (<10%) after just one year."

In writing about fecal incontinence among prostate cancer patients, the National Center for Biotechnology Information (NCBI) at the US National Library of Medicine in Bethesda, Maryland, identified 994 articles on the subject for consideration, with 213 "selected for full article review of which 40 were selected" for the final review.[19] The review results show that the "incidence of fecal incontinence following radiotherapy for prostate cancer varied from 1.6% to 58%," an amazingly wide range. The report stated that the cause of "fecal incontinence was not entirely clear," but it is most likely due to injury to the muscular nerves in the anal-rectal area.

A variety of interventions may be considered to control fecal incontinence. According to MedicineWeb, they include the following:

- Increasing the strength of the pelvic floor muscles
- Use of Kegel exercises (the same as used to control urinary incontinence)
- Use of electrical stimulation

Biofeedback "is often used to help retrain the anal sphincters and have the patient appreciate the sensation of rectal fullness that comes just before the need to defecate."

Surgery may be attempted to repair the muscles of the pelvic floor, including the external anal sphincter; as a last resort, a colostomy may be performed, where the colon is diverted through the abdominal wall to empty into a removable bag.

POTENTIALLY TRAGIC CONSEQUENCES

While prostate cancer may not be as deadly as it once was, a new study suggests that any diagnosis of the disease carries risks.

Researchers from Harvard University and Sweden's Karolinska Institute studied data accumulated from four million Swedish men over the age of thirty and found that even the diagnosis of prostate cancer increased the risks for fatal heart problems eleven times and suicide by eight times in the week after diagnosis. This was the finding for 4 percent of the sample, which totaled over 160,000.[20]

These findings demonstrate that:

- It is important to inform men of the physical changes that they may experience.
- It is at least equally important that these men understand that there are ways of managing those changes. It should also be emphasized that many men have overcome these challenges and gone on to lead positive and productive lives.

"Stress can be an important trigger for physiologic reactions, including increased risk of cardiovascular disease," said Dr. Meir Stampfer, professor of nutrition and epidemiology at the Harvard School of Public Health. "The diagnosis of cancer also can cause high enough stress to see a noticeable increase in both heart disease and suicide."

"This study is certainly a wakeup call that there are other issues . . . that somebody could be at increased cardiovascular risk or increased suicide risk," said Bruce Trock, an epidemiologist in the Department of Urology at Johns Hopkins. "The lesson [of the study] is more for

About Harold's Prostate Situation

Harold was a Harvard Medical School graduate whose life was rewarding both personally and professionally. Harold had the joy of an "ideal marriage" to Margaret, who was an accomplished academic and had loyally supported and encouraged Harold for more than fifty years.

Then, in his seventy-third year, Harold discovered blood in his urine. Concerned, but not alarmed, Harold notified his personal physician and long-time friend, who proceeded cautiously. The initial testing began with the usual PSA blood test followed by a digital rectal exam.

The results showed that Harold had metastatic prostate cancer. First came the radical prostatectomy, then a regime of radiation therapy. But the PSA remained obstinate and challenging, so Harold's oncology team set about a regimen of strong Androgen Deprivation Therapy, or ADT. By that time, Harold was experiencing urinary incontinence, and fecal incontinence was developing. Yet, the ADT had succeeded in stopping the cancer growth.

While the treatment was medically successful, patient Harold was deteriorating. The increasing annoyance of his incontinence was complicated by bone pain, fatigue, and depression. Not only had he fully retired from his position at a major teaching university, but he also was mentally disengaging from the events and people around him, those who had admired and supported him and his work for decades.

During the nearly four years Harold lived with his prostate cancer, the pain in his bones increased, the daily challenges of just living became more difficult, and the constant attention to his bodily functions robbed him of any remaining sense of a good quality of life. Indeed, life had become one continuing and seemingly overwhelmingly hellish ordeal.

Although successful medically—since the hormone therapy kept the cancer from spreading—the treatment created an unacceptably poor quality of life for Harold.

After dwelling on the state of his existence and the future he foresaw for himself, Harold wrote a farewell note and then emailed it to friends and colleagues. In his letter, Harold stated that he was terminating treatment and was preparing to die, seeing this as the better alternative to living. He proceeded as planned and died a few weeks later.

physicians, that when they give out a diagnosis of prostate cancer, they should be thinking about this."

Sometimes reality is simply too real, too much to take. And this is a fact that all individuals who deal with prostate cancer patients should come to grips with. The case of Harold, the Boston doctor who developed prostate cancer (and whose case was mentioned earlier in chapter 19), is dramatically illustrative of one such outcome.

IN OUR OPINION. . .

To say prostate cancer is a "life changing" event is certainly not an exaggeration. By now, you have read how prostate cancer will change your physical body, how your body functions on daily basis, how you relate to your sexual partner, and perhaps even how long you will live. Those are, indeed, "life-changing" alterations in anyone's world.

To ask how long recovery will take is an unanswerable question because you never recover: you change.

In all likelihood, your attitude changes, your physiology changes, and your values change. In a sense, you are a different man in what appears to be the same body, but that has changed, too.

In addition to the significant physiological changes wrought by prostate cancer treatment, one oncologist related a patient's story that explains the psychological changes. He described a Boston-area police chief—a big, burly guy with a thick Boston accent. Some months after the end of his treatment and during a routine follow-up visit, the police chief explained to his oncologist that, "You won't believe how much I've changed. How much my emotions have changed. It used to be that nothing affected me. On the force for thirty-seven years, I'd seen everything. I thought there was nothing new."

"But now," the chief said, "it's the damnedest thing. You tell me a story about a little baby who's screaming and crying and one of my guys—or a fireman—rescues the kid from a burning house, and I start to cry big crocodile tears. Stories like that really affect me. I'm so sympathetic now. So emotional.".

And that was a good outcome resulting from treatment. We all should be so lucky.

21

Aids for Your Return to Sexual Activity

What's sexually normal for a twenty-four-year-old man is quite different from what is normal for his sixty-year-old father. Therefore, "normal" is a fluid and a very personal term; its definition changes according to your age and experiences.

Whatever your definition of "normal" is, however, you can be assured that after prostate cancer treatment, you will not be the same "normal" person you were. New prosthetic-type interventions have been developed that seek to disguise the results of your prostate cancer experiences, but they only mask the real facts. You ARE different after treatment for prostate cancer. Period. You are beginning a period of the "new normal."

Given that fact, aids for helping you cope with this "new normal" can help restore the old you, even though you are not that person.

CANCER TREATMENT SIDE EFFECTS

Treatments for prostate cancer clearly have serious implications for the conduct of a man's life, yet despite the widespread existence of prostate cancer, little progress seems to have been made in developing effective rehabilitation practices for the men who have undergone one or more prostate cancer treatments.

Johns Hopkins University reports the follow results from different prostate cancer treatments:[1]

- One year following a nerve-sparing prostatectomy, 40 percent to 50 percent will regain pretreatment functional sexual ability.

- Two years following a nerve-sparing prostatectomy, 30 percent to 60 percent will regain pretreatment functional sexual ability.

Johns Hopkins warns that these rates vary widely depending on the surgeon and the extent to which he can successfully perform the "nerve-sparing" operation, and it further offers the following statistics.

- About 25 percent to 50 percent of men who undergo brachytherapy (seeds) will experience erectile dysfunction versus about 50 percent who have external beam radiation.
- "After two to three years, few men will see much of an improvement and occasionally these numbers worsen over time."
- "Men who undergo procedures not designed to minimize side effects and/or those whose treatments are administered by physicians who are not proficient in the procedures will fare worse."
- Harvard University's 2009 "Report on Prostate Cancer," has similar statistics, which show that: 30 percent to 70 percent of men who undergo radical prostatectomy or external beam radiation therapy will develop impotence after treatment.[2]
- 30 percent to 50 percent of men who opt for brachytherapy will develop impotence after treatment.

While the problems resulting from various prostate cancer treatments range from ED to incontinence, at least some victories have been achieved in addressing the ED problem. Each of the three primary prostate cancer treatments, however—surgery, radiation, and hormone therapy—has its own set of erectile dysfunction aftereffects.

- A radical prostatectomy removes the prostate gland and—in the process—nerves, blood vessels, and muscles may be damaged. That is why your surgeon will tell you that he "will try to preserve as many nerves as possible" during surgery.
- A radical prostatectomy may take one of three forms: traditional open surgery, the less invasive laparoscopic surgery, or robot-assisted techniques.
- Depending on the degree to which the tissues surrounding your prostate gland are preserved, you may not be able to have an erection for a month or longer—or, perhaps, forever—following surgery.

- Radiation therapy damages the nerves near your prostate and can affect your ability to have an erection. "Some men start having erectile dysfunction six months or more after their radiation therapy. If this happens, the erectile dysfunction usually does not improve," UCLA says. Additionally, if you can achieve an orgasm, you will notice that you ejaculate less semen. Over time, the amount of semen will diminish, and you will have "dry ejaculations."
- Hormone therapy reduces the amount of testosterone your body produces rather than damage tissues around the prostate. While the side effects of hormone therapy are different from man to man, the usual complications include a loss of interest in sex, erectile dysfunction, and/or the inability to reach an orgasm.

While ED receives the greatest notice in the discussion of prostate cancer recovery, other outcomes can be as devastating—or more so—than erectile dysfunction.

Yet, there is at least some hope!

One more comment on the subject of "lifestyle-limiting conditions." We believe that men—and their characteristic silence—may be their own worst enemies in any effort to light a fire under medical researchers regarding prostate cancer rehabilitation.

Previously, we noted a joint research report by CancerCare and UsTOO International that stated: "97% of the respondents believed there was a need to help patients recognize these symptoms [of depression and anxiety] and find treatment for them." While there was near unanimity about the perceived "need," few actually did or said anything about that unfulfilled need.

We also noted, and believe it is worth repeating:

Men tend not to seek out help for psycho-social issues—notably less often than women do. This is borne out by survey results that suggest men with prostate cancer would benefit from support groups, yet they seldom attend them, and other data shows that women outnumber men by three-to-one in cancer support groups.

We believe that if men, who tend to be such mouthy leaders in some areas, would become more vocal about the need for better prostate cancer treatment, counseling, and rehabilitation, then positive developments would occur. We can only hope!

ORAL TREATMENTS

Oral medications, which were first developed in 1998, are popular with men affected by ED, with or without prostate treatments. They can begin working in about half an hour and last up to thirty-six hours, although eight hours is more realistic. They relax the penis muscles, which allows an increased blood flow, thus stimulating an erection.

Oral medications for ED are not for use by all men, especially those with heart problems who are taking medications for angina or alpha-blockers. However, among those men who do take oral medications, about three-quarters of them get positive results.[3]

FDA-approved drugs for ED include Viagra™ (sildenafil), Cialis™ (tadalafil), and Levitra™ (vardenafil), which work by blocking an enzyme in the penis called Phosphodiesterase V (PDE V). This improves blood flow to the penis (as mentioned above) and allows a natural chemical in the body to initiate, produce, and maintain an erection.

Harvard University reported that in a very limited study of seventy-six participants in 2008, "27% of men in the sildenafil group reported satisfactory erectile function, but only 4% in the placebo group."

Yet another study in 2008 (with a group of 628 men) using the drug vardenafil (or Levitra™) resulted in satisfactory erectile function in the range of 48 percent to 54 percent. It was reported as well that for these medications to be effective, patients needed sexual stimulation and foreplay to initiate an erection.

VACUUM DEVICES

Vacuum devices are a noninvasive way to treat ED and are available in both prescription (recommended) and nonprescription forms. The cylindrical device is placed over the penis and then mechanically creates a vacuum in the cylinder of the pump chamber; the erection is maintained using constriction rings. One manufacturer, Advanced Urological Care, P.C., described the process as such: "After the penis and constriction rings are coated with water-soluble lubricant and the rings are loaded onto the cylinder base, the cylinder is placed over the penis with the base held firmly against the pubis to maintain a seal. The pump is then activated to slowly create negative pressure, or a vacuum, inside the cylinder, which draws blood into the corpora cavernosa, producing an erection.

Once the penis is engorged, the constriction band is pulled from the cylinder onto the base of the penis. The negative pressure is released through a valve, and the cylinder is removed. It takes an average of several minutes to create an erection through this procedure.

The erection produced by vacuum devices, however, differs significantly from a normal erection: the penile skin temperature is lower and the appearance bluer. The veins of the penis appear distended, and penile circumference is increased. In addition, the penis may pivot at the base, requiring the patient to stabilize the penis during intercourse.

INJECTIONS

Alprostadil is an FDA-approved drug that is injected directly into the penis to trigger an erection. It is reported to have an 85 percent success rate–if the user and his partner don't mind the injection preparation. "Penile injection is the most effective type of ED treatment for men who can't take oral treatment," according to Dr. Nelson Bennett, a urologist at the Lahey Clinic in Burlington, Massachusetts.[4]

The injection therapy works when a needle is used to inject medication directly into the base or side of the penis. The medication allows blood to flow into the penis, creating an erection in five to ten minutes. A burning sensation is the possible side effect; an erection that lasts more than four hours requires medical attention. A patient or his partner must learn to perform a penile injection each time a man wishes an erection, which will last from about 30 minutes to an hour—or up to orgasm.[5] Alprostadil in two medications—Coverlet™ or EDEX™—dilates the arteries of the penis and allows an inflow of blood, with erection occurring from five to fifteen minutes after injection.

A patient or his partner must learn to perform a penile injection each time a man wishes an erection, which will last from about thirty minutes to an hour—or up to orgasm.[6] Patients who have tried the injection method complain that while they "have plenty of intent," they gave up on the execution. Some spouses say that the injection approach is a "turn off" and is like "flogging a dead horse." Obviously, not every patient finds injections successful or even satisfactory. One user explained it this way: "When I first did a penile injection, it worked, but my wife was so turned off by it and even the idea made her disinterested. So, it became useless for enabling sexual intercourse between us."

Fortunately, if a man or his partner resists an injection, Alprostadil comes in a suppository that is used by inserting it into the urethra, as directed by your doctor. This FDA-approved drug alternative goes by the name of MUSE (which stands for: Medicated Urethral System for Erection) and is absorbed through the urethra, then distributed into surrounding tissues. An erection is produced in about ten minutes when the blood vessels enlarge and blood flows into them, causing the penis to harden. Side effects may be an aching, burning, or redness as well as minor bleeding.

IMPLANTS

Nothing about prostate cancer is easy: deciding on implant surgery and "achieving optimum results depends on selection of a penile device/ manufacturer best suited for each patient," as well as a thorough knowledge of the patient's history and personal behavioral characteristics. The characteristics and variables the medical team, as well as the patient, must consider include:

- Overall health of patient
- Age of the patient and his partner or spouse
- Patient's life expectancy
- Overall penile size
- Overall size of scrotum
- History of previous penile implants
- Whether or not the penis is circumcised
- Ratio between crus (buried) and pendulous penis
- History of kidney transplants or major pelvic surgery
- Presence or absence of penile curvature or fibrosis
- Presence of a colostomy, ideal conduit or neo-bladder
- Ratio between penile length and size of scrotum
- Presence of penile shaft or penis atrophy or deformity (Peyronie's disease)

- Previous peripheral vascular surgery (femoral to femoral artery bypass)
- Previous abdominal surgery (bladder, prostate, and colon) and type (open versus laparoscopy or robot)

The Mayo Clinic suggests three possible types of implants: three-piece inflatable, two-piece inflatable, and the Semirigid rod. The clinic notes on its website, "When choosing which type of penile implant is right for you, consider your personal preference and your medical history. Your doctor might suggest one type of design over another based on your age, risk of infection, and health conditions, injuries or medical treatments you've had in the past."

For each of the three types, the clinic lists the pros and cons:[7]

1. Three-piece inflatable

   Pros

   - Creates the most natural, rigid erection.
   - Provides flaccidity when deflated.

   Cons

   - Has more parts that could malfunction than do other implants.
   - Requires a reservoir inside the abdomen.

2. Two-piece inflatable

   Pros

   - Provides flaccidity when deflated.

   Cons

   - Is mechanically more complicated than is a semirigid implant.
   - Provides less-firm erections than does a three-piece implant.

3. Semirigid rod

   Pros

   - Has a low chance of malfunction due to the small number of parts.

- Is easy to use for those with limited mental or manual dexterity.

Cons

- Results in a penis that is always slightly rigid.
- Puts constant pressure on the inside of the penis, which can cause injury.
- Can be difficult to conceal under clothing.

IN OUR OPINION. . .

Especially in the case of erectile dysfunction, the cliché that "reality is what you perceive to be real" has special meaning. And the reality for prostate cancer patients is that their sexual ability is not what it used to be, and never will be.

While we believe that oncology researchers have attempted to lessen the blow of dealing with erectile dysfunction, the fact remains that having conventional sex will never be the same again. Since physiology is likely to be an unfortunate victim in dealing with prostate cancer, the psychological aspects of our lives must therefore become more prominent. Research studies show that:

Depression was 56% and was significantly higher than in men in [a] control group with benign prostatic hyperplasia. . . . For those men who are particularly bothered by sexual dysfunction, the first step should be a consultation with a urologist who specializes in male sexual dysfunction. Sex therapy with a trained therapist may help a man express the feelings engendered by this dysfunction, and also to help a couple learn alternative ways of sharing sexual intimacy.[8]

Even with the assistance of an experienced sex therapist, however, one fact remains: your sexual life—to say nothing about your life as a whole—will never again be the same as you remember it.

Section 7

PROSTATE CANCER DEVELOPMENT

22

What Is My Prostate Gland, and Why Is It Important?

Your prostate gland is an important part of your daily life. Weighing about one ounce, it is often referred to as "walnut-sized" mass and located in your pelvis and has the primary role of providing semen. Without your prostate gland, you would not be able to generate normal amounts of semen—and fathering a child would be impossible. The gland's muscles also help propel the semen, which is about one-third fluid that is excreted by the prostate gland.

Therefore, the prostate helps perform an important role in urination and ejaculation—the two activities directly affected when a man is treated for prostate cancer. While the prostate gland is well located for assisting in ejaculation, its proximity to the urethra can be a liability if the gland swells or grows, interfering with urination.

Just because you have prostate problems—trouble urinating—does not mean you have prostate cancer. Rather, you could have prostatitis (inflammation of the prostate) or BPH (benign prostatic hypertrophy), common among men over fifty years old.

By the time a man reaches age forty, his prostate might have grown from the size of a walnut to the size of an apricot and weigh about three-fourths of an ounce.

The prostate is prone to developing disorders, three of which are not uncommon.

1. Prostatitis is an inflammation of the prostate, which is sometimes caused by an infection. It can be treated with antibiotics.
2. An enlarged prostate is called benign prostatic hypertrophy, or BPH, which affects many men over fifty. Symptoms of BPH

include difficulty in urination, which tends to increase as a man ages. *Medical News Today* says that BPH can "affect almost all men aged 50 or over—yet surgery can treat BPH."[1]

3. Prostate cancer is the second most common form of cancer in men (after skin cancer). Surgery, radiation, hormone therapy, and chemotherapy are used to treat prostate cancer. Some men and their doctors, however, choose to delay treatment, which is called "watchful waiting."

"Most of the fluid in semen is made up of secretions from male reproductive organs. Semen contains citric acid, free amino acids, fructose, enzymes, phosphorylcholine, prostaglandin, potassium, and zinc," according to Medical Life Sciences.[2]

One component of the prostate fluid is the enzyme called the prostate-specific antigen (PSA), and measurement of an elevated PSA level in your blood may be an indicator of the presence of cancer. It should be noted that only between 13 percent and 33 percent of the fluid is actually produced by the prostate gland.

- 46 percent to 80 percent of the fluid is produced by the seminal vesicles.
- 5 percent is from the testicles and epididymis.
- 2 percent to 5 percent is from Bulbourethral and urethral glands.

Conditions that indicate your prostate may not be operating properly and should compel you to see your doctor for a professional opinion include the following.[3]

- Frequent urination
- Urination that burns
- Difficulty with starting urine flow
- Weak flow, or "dribbling"
- Blood in the urine

IN OUR OPINION. . .

The prostate gland is small but mighty. We believe that it should be considered an extremely important part of a man's body given its role in his daily life and reproductive activities.

To summarize its importance in a man's life: "The prostate's most important function is the production of a fluid that, together with sperm cells from the testicles and fluids from other glands, makes up semen." [4]

This fluid helps sperm travel more easily, thus increasing the likelihood of successfully fertilizing an egg. The alkaline nature of the fluid helps counteract the acidity of the vagina and protect the sperm from damage.

Because the prostate is such an integral part of men being men, we believe that its care is underrated—until something goes wrong. Therefore, while you can't control your culture, race, father's prostate history, or the part of the world where you are raised, you can control your diet, your physical condition, and much of your medical awareness.

The following chapter deals with managing your lifestyle so that you have a chance to control that which you can actually control.

How Did I Develop Prostate Cancer?

As men age, their likelihood of developing prostate cancer increases. And the older you get, the greater the likelihood that you will develop an enlarged prostate or even prostate cancer. If prostate cancer runs in your family, you also have an increased chance of developing the disease.

Black men are most susceptible to developing prostate cancer, followed by whites and Asians. Your susceptibility increases beginning at about age forty.

A normal prostate at age forty is the size of a walnut; by your mid-fifties, it is the size of an apricot, and that of a lemon by your seventies. A growing prostate can signal cancer.

Based on historical statistics, about 60 percent of men over age sixty-five can expect to develop an enlarged prostate. You also have a greater chance of developing prostate cancer if you are an overweight, balding, older, black man who indulges in grilled meats and smokes and whose father had the disease.

One basic answer to the question, "How did I develop prostate cancer" is simply that you're getting older. While somewhat glib, the fact is that no one is exactly certain what causes prostate cancer. Age, race, genetics, diet, even height, some contend, are surely contributors to development of prostate cancer. Thus, your whole physiology determines your chances of developing prostate cancer.

One particularly interesting finding is that patterned hair loss is associated with an increased risk of fatal prostate cancer, according to the survey results of a National Health and Nutrition Examination (NHNES) reported in 2016 in the *American Journal of Epidemiology*. NHNES surveyed 4,316 men ages twenty-five to seventy-four with no prior cancer diagnosis and arrived at the following research results, among others.

- Any baldness was associated with a 56 percent higher risk of fatal prostate cancer.
- Moderate balding was specifically associated with an 83 percent higher risk of prostate cancer.

While this is only one study addressing a possible relationship between baldness and prostate cancer, it is worth noting since patterned hair loss is dependent on androgen as well as genetic predisposition. You might say, as George Orwell wrote in his prophetic book *Animal Farm*: "All animals are equal, but some animals are more equal than others."[1]

The Prostate Cancer Foundation (PCF) says that six key factors influence your likelihood of developing prostate cancer. They are:

- Age
- Genetics and family history
- Race
- Nationality
- Lifestyle and diet

Other risk factors may include height, nationality, and even ejaculation frequency.[2]

Let's delve into the details.

AGE

"The older you get one thing is certain, the more likely you are to be diagnosed with prostate cancer," according to the PCF. The rates of prostate cancer diagnosis based on age are the following:

- 1 in 10,000 for men under age forty
- 1 in 39 for men ages forty to fifty-nine
- 1 in 14 for men ages sixty to sixty-nine

In fact, nearly 60 percent of all prostate cancers are diagnosed in men over the age of sixty-five. As indicated by the rates of diagnosis, age is the biggest—but not the only—risk factor for prostate cancer in men. While it's relatively rare among men younger than forty, the chance of having prostate cancer rises rapidly among men over age fifty. Only skin cancer is more common among men than prostate cancer, the second leading cause of death overall among men after heart disease.

More than half of men in their sixties suffer from a growth of the prostate called benign prostatic hyperplasia (BPH), which is a nonmalignant enlarged prostate, according to the Ohio State University Medical Center. BPH is common and cannot be prevented: age and a family history of BPH are two factors that increase your chances of developing it. Since your prostate surrounds part of your urethra, when it becomes enlarged, it can limit your ability to urinate. This symptom is typical of BPH and tends to occur when you are fifty or older, but it can start earlier. By the time you're seventy or eighty, your chance of suffering BPH jumps to 90 percent.

The American Cancer Society reports that:[3]

- 80 percent of men develop an enlarged prostate.
- ~90 percent of men over the age of eighty-five have BPH.
- ~30 percent of men find their symptoms bothersome.

GENETICS AND FAMILY HISTORY

In addition to the age connection, the PCF says that the genes for prostate cancer "can run in families. . . . About 5% to 10% of all prostate cancers diagnosed are hereditary," according to New York's Memorial Sloan-Kettering Cancer Center.

"Men who have a relative with prostate cancer are twice as likely to develop the disease, while those with 2 or more relatives are nearly 4 times as likely to be diagnosed. The risk is even higher if the affected family members were diagnosed before age 65," according to the PCF, which also said that men may also be at increased risk of prostate cancer if they have a strong family history of other cancers, such as breast, ovarian, colon, or pancreatic cancer. This is because members of the same family have many genes in common, and "there may be multiple genetic factors that contribute to the overall risk of prostate cancer in a family," says the Prostate Cancer Foundation.

And Sloan-Kettering says that "Family history is the strongest risk factor for prostate cancer. . . . A man who has one close relative with prostate cancer (for example, a father or a brother) has twice the likelihood of developing prostate cancer as a man with no family history of the disease."[4] If you have two close male relatives who have or have had prostate cancer, then your "lifetime risk of developing prostate cancer is increased five-fold."

Scientists have recently discovered the common thread among male family members is a gene called BRCA2, which seems to increase a man's risk for prostate cancer. Not only does BRCA2 suppress cell growth, according to the National Cancer Institute of the NIH, but certain mutations of the inherited gene (on Chromosome 13) indicate that a man has a higher risk of prostate cancer. When it appears among women, they have an increased chance of developing ovarian and breast cancer. "The BRCA2 gene provides instructions for making a protein that acts as a tumor suppressor. Tumor suppressor proteins help prevent cells from growing and dividing too rapidly or in an uncontrolled way," says the NIH.[5] "Investigators are now working to determine to what extent this and other mutations play a role in causing the disease," Sloan-Kettering reports. Such understanding may lead to improved methods of identifying "men who are at increased risk, and [it] could also lead to the development of new treatments."

England's Oxford University says that "tall men have a heightened risk of dying from aggressive prostate cancer," according to a report in *The Independent* of London.[6] "British scientists found no association between height and overall prostate cancer risk, but [did find] a strong link with high-grade, deadly tumors."

RACE

Prostate cancer occurs more frequently among African American and Caribbean men of African ancestry than among white males. Indeed, African American men are more than twice as likely to die of prostate cancer than white men.

Table 23.1. Percent Distributions of PCa

Asian-Pacific	8.6%
Hispanic-Latino	15.7%
Non-Hispanic White	18.0%
Native American	18.7%
All Races	19.1 %
Non-Hispanic Black	38.7%

However, an "unexpected" finding emerged in pooled data from nine phase III trials of chemotherapy for advanced disease, according to a February 2019 report in the *Journal of Clinical Oncology*. The study included 8,820 men, with 85 percent white, 6 percent black, 5 percent Asian, and 4 percent of unknown ethnicity. It showed that "black and white men with metastatic castration-resistant prostate cancer treated with standard chemotherapy in phase 3 clinical trials had similar overall survival."

Nonetheless, "while prostate cancer deaths have been reduced by more than 50% in the last two decades, the reality is still worse for African American men," writes the Prostate Cancer Foundation, adding that African American men are 76 percent more likely to be diagnosed with prostate cancer than are Caucasian men. "Although scientists do not yet understand why prostate cancer incidence and death rates are higher among African American men, it is widely believed that a combination of genetic differences, lifestyle and nutrition habits, and access to medical care may all play a role in the statistics."[7]

"The bottom line is, in a sense, that African American men with advanced prostate cancer need to get to an oncologist and ideally need to get on a clinical trial," according to Dr. Richard Schilsky, who is the chief medical officer of the American Society of Clinical Oncologists. "And if they do, their outcomes are every bit as good as Caucasian men."[8]

According to Dr. Quoc-Dien Trinh, codirector of the Dana-Farber/Brigham and Women's Prostate Cancer Center in Boston, however, "Black men with riskier prostate cancers may be less likely than their white counterparts to get aggressive treatment that can give them the best survival odds."[9] "Black patients are also more likely to be diagnosed when tumors are more advanced and more difficult to treat," implying that medical recognition of the cancer was discovered in its later stage of development, according to a report in the online publication *European Urology* (August 2, 2017).

"For decades, African-American men have had the highest prostate cancer incidence rate of any racial-ethnic group in the world. At 261.9 new cases per 100,000 in 1993, their rate is two-thirds higher than whites and more than twice as high as rates for Asian-Americans," according to the *Journal of the National Cancer Institute*.[10] While prostate cancer does occur less often in Asian American and Hispanic or Latino males, the reasons for such racial and ethnic differences remain unclear to medical researchers.[11] Investigators at the Southwest Oncology Group speculate, however, that "differences in tumor biology associated with race or ethnicity, such as the way the body metabolizes chemotherapy drugs, might make cancers in African Americans more aggressive or resistant to treatment."[12]

NATIONALITY

The incidence of prostate cancer varies significantly around the world. "The highest rates are in Australia and New Zealand, Northern and Western Europe and North America," according to World Cancer Research Fund of the American Institute for Cancer Research,[13] which also noted that the incidence of prostate cancer in the United States was ten times the levels in the Far East. The lowest rates of occurrence are in poorer countries and those where the populations characteristically have diets that are less dominated by red meat, which include China, India, Japan, and Singapore. Death rates from prostate cancer mirror the incidence statistics.

LIFESTYLE AND DIET

The Continuous Update Project of the World Cancer Research Fund conducted what it called the most rigorous and systematic global analysis of the scientific research currently available on diet, weight, physical activity, and prostate cancer, and it concluded that there is "strong evidence that being overweight or obese increases the risk of advanced prostate cancer."

Obesity is largely a Western problem and one that is, unfortunately, strongly associated with the United States. This is borne out when one looks at the changes in individual health of people migrating from low-fat countries like Japan to high-fat countries like the United States.

For example, in his book *Diet and Prostate Cancer,* author Danish Mazhar notes that, "when migrants from a low-risk country such as Japan move to the United States, a high-risk nation, their prostate cancer incidence and mortality become several-fold higher than native Japanese counterparts."[14]

He adds that:

> A positive correlation exists between the number of years since migration to the United States and cancer risk. Diet is one of the environmental factors suspected to play a role in the etiology [science dealing with disease causes] of prostate cancer. High dietary intakes of dairy products, meat, and fat, and low consumption of tomatoes, selenium, and vitamins D and E have all been associated with higher prostate cancer risk.

The *2017 Annual Report on Prostate Cancer* published by Harvard University cites another common culprit for negative health conditions: smoking. "Declines in prostate cancer mortality rates appear to parallel declines in smoking prevalence at the population level," according to a report by the Centers for Disease Control and Prevention in Atlanta. "This study suggests that declines in prostate cancer mortality rates may be a beneficial effect of reduced smoking in the population."[15]

The CDC report showed the following linkages during the period 1999 through 2010.

- Smoking in California declined by 3.5 percent per year, and prostate cancer mortality rates declined by 2.5 percent per year.
- In Kentucky, smoking declined by 3.0 percent per year, and prostate cancer mortality rates declined by 3.5 percent per year.
- In Maryland, smoking declined by 3.0 percent per year, and prostate cancer mortality rates declined by 3.5 percent per year.
- In Utah, smoking declined by 3.5 percent per year, and prostate cancer mortality rates declined by 2.1 percent per year.

IN OUR OPINION. . .

Perhaps the mother's admonition that "You are what you eat (or smoke)" has never been more bluntly associated with a human condition than in the case of prostate cancer.

It seems that a life filled with "healthful" food, a reasonable amount of exercise, and a temperate lifestyle can contribute to your avoiding prostate cancer. That is, of course, if you are not too tall, too fat, black, live in a food-gorging Western country, and don't have any relatives with a history of prostate cancer. Other than that, you're probably just fine.

On a more serious note, the next chapter provides specifics about a healthful diet, and that's important with or without prostate cancer. We also present some dietary strategies that claim to mitigate the impact, or even the spread, of prostate cancer. Read on!

Can Prostate Cancer Be Prevented?

While there is no cure for prostate cancer, but paying attention to your lifestyle, diet, and the amount of exercise you engage in may be helpful in preventing—or slowing—the rate of prostate cancer development.

In short, you must pay attention to your diet, weight, and exercise. Those are the same recommendations that you hear almost daily, and they just may work. At least, they're worth a try.

Some things in life you can't change, such as your parents and the culture that you grow up in. However, there are many aspects of your life that you can change, and those changes may help you avoid prostate cancer, or at least forestall its early onset or restrict its development.

The Mayo Clinic is pretty blunt about it: "There's no proven prostate cancer prevention strategy. But you may reduce your risk of prostate cancer by making healthy choices, such as exercising and eating a healthy diet."[1]

They recommend that you

1. Eat a healthful diet.
2. Exercise and maintain a healthy weight.
3. Sleep well and get enough rest.

The Prostate Cancer Foundation (PCF) agrees, and says that, "42% of cancer cases are thought to be preventable with the right lifestyle changes, including but limited to HPV vaccinations, quitting smoking, and reducing obesity. It is never too late to develop a personalized wellness plan."[2] While most of that statement is readily understood, perhaps the mention of HPV is not. The Centers for Disease Control and Prevention explains it simply:

> Nearly all sexually active people will get human papillomavirus (HPV) at some time in their life if they don't get the HPV vaccine. Although most HPV infections go away on their own without causing problems, HPV can cause genital warts, or cancer. Getting vaccinated against HPV can help prevent these health problems. . . . HPV is a very common virus that can be spread from one person to another person through anal, vaginal, or oral sex, or through other close skin-to-skin touching during sexual activity. More than 79 million Americans, most in their late teens and early 20s, are infected with HPV. Nearly all sexually active people who do not get the HPV vaccine get infected with HPV at some point in their lives.[3]

CHOOSE A HEALTHFUL DIET

While there's no concrete proof that diet influences the onset or the development of prostate cancer, there is "some evidence that choosing a healthy diet that's low in fat and full of fruits and vegetables may contribute to a lower risk of prostate cancer." Such a diet, the Mayo Clinic says, is characterized by reduction in fatty food choices such as meats, nuts, cooking and salad oils, and dairy products like milk and cheese. The clinic says that in some studies, "Men who ate the highest amount of fat each day had an increased risk of prostate cancer." And even if this effort does not prevent prostate cancer, it will go a long way toward helping you keep a desirable weight and help the condition of your heart.

You mother told you to "eat your vegetables," and she was right! Mother Mayo suggests to "eat more fat from plants than from animals." That means reducing the amount of red meat, lard, and butter that you consume, and using olive oil instead of butter. Increase the amount of fruits and vegetables you eat because they are loaded with vitamins and nutrients that are believed to reduce the risk of prostate cancer.

The American Cancer Society notes that "several studies have suggested that diets high in certain vegetables—including tomatoes, cruciferous vegetables (cabbage, broccoli, and cauliflower), beans, soy, and other legumes—or fish may be linked with a lower risk of prostate cancer, especially more advanced cancers."[4]

Eat more fish (such as salmon, tuna, and herring) because they contain omega-3 fatty acids, which have been linked to a reduced prostate cancer risk. Flaxseed is also a way to add omega-3s to your diet.

You can reduce your consumption of dairy products by cutting back on such items as milk, cheese, and yogurt. While study results "have been mixed and the risks associated with dairy products are thought to be small," some would say that every step counts in the battle against prostate cancer.

Although there are conflicting beliefs about the value of any one collection of dietary items that collectively help prevent prostate cancer, there is something of a consensus about what constitutes a healthful diet. The PCF suggests a nine-point diet to help "prevent" prostate cancer. If you are reading this, however, *preventing* prostate cancer is likely now history. Nonetheless, the PCF recommendations track with other sources of advice for prostate cancer patients' diets and include the following nine points.

1. Drink extra virgin olive oil at the rate of four tablespoons per day.
2. Men should eat tofu because soy's high concentration of phytoestrogens—for example, naturally occurring estrogen—can ward off prostate cancer (although it can cause increased risk of breast cancer and possible infertility in women).
3. Reduce stress in your life.
4. Smoking makes no sense at any time and after a diagnosis of prostate cancer makes metastases worse. A May 2008 study published in *JAMA Oncology* indicates that "men who smoke during localized prostate cancer treatment are more likely to recur or develop metastasis."
5. The Prostate Cancer Foundation says that lycopene in cooked tomatoes "has long been known to ward off prostate cancer" and that Sofrito (from the verb soffriggere: to stir fry) as a tomato-based sauce is a good source. It is used as a cooking base in many cultures, from Spain to Puerto Rico.
6. While tomatoes contain vitamins A and C—important for immunity and cell repair—their lycopene "can protect cells from the damage caused by chemicals called free radicals. This makes

tomatoes potentially a great food to fight cancer," according to the PCF.[5]

7. Drink green tea because it helps prevent the angiogenesis process, by which tumor cells encourage blood vessel growth to feed themselves. "Green tea inhibits cellular ability to recruit new blood vessels," and thus limits tumor growth, say a PCF publication.[6]

8. Three or more cups of coffee a day "can cut your risk of prostate cancer in half," believes the PCF.

9. "Vigorous exercise and other healthy habits may cut a man's chances of developing prostate cancer by a full 68%," according to the foundation.

10. Under the classification of "How to eat red meat without killing yourself," the foundation recommends that you always eat grass-fed beef and never eat charred meat (so much for the wonderful aroma and flavor of a steak seared on the grill).

MAINTAIN A HEALTHFUL WEIGHT

"Men who are obese—a body mass index (BMI) of 30 or higher—may have an increased risk of prostate cancer," Mayo says. Losing weight means cutting the number of calories you consume daily. Studies have shown that men who exercise regularly may have a reduced risk of prostate cancer, writes Mayo, and exercise is also good for your heart. A few simple changes in your behavior can make an important difference in your health and the way you feel, for instance, taking the stairs instead of taking the elevator, walking the dog, or just walking yourself.

Food or nutritional intake clearly has an impact on the way we feel and our bodies' abilities to deal with the likes of prostate cancer. Author Dr. Pier Paolo Pandolfi, who is the HMS George C. Reisman Professor of Medicine at Beth Israel Deaconess in Boston, wrote:

> The progression of cancer to the metastatic stage represents a pivotal event that influences patient outcomes and the therapeutic options available to patients. Our data provide a strong genetic foundation for the mechanisms underlying metastatic progression, and we also demonstrated how environmental factors can boost these mechanisms to promote progression from primary to advanced metastatic cancer.[7]

Pandolfi noted that the "findings also helped solve a long-standing scientific puzzle. For years, researchers had difficulty modeling metastatic prostate cancer in mice," so he asked, 'What do our mice eat?'" It turned out the mice ate a vegetable-based chow, essentially a low-fat vegan diet that bore little resemblance to that of the average American male. When Pandolfi and colleagues increased the levels of saturated fats, the kind found in fast food cheeseburgers and fries, in the animals' diet, the mice developed aggressive, metastatic tumors.

Their research could help humans by starving tumors of fat, "either with the fat-blocking drug or through diet. . . . The data are tremendously actionable, and they surely will convince you to change your lifestyle," Pandolfi said.[8]

Epidemiologists also note that many types of cancer, including metastatic cancers, are much higher in the United States than in other parts of the world, where lower-fat diets are common. For instance, they note that while 10 percent of Asian men develop prostate cancer, 40 percent of American men develop the disease. Emphasizing the dietary relationship to the disease, the same researcher notes that when Asian men immigrate to the United States, their rate of prostate cancer rises to the American level of 40 percent.

(An interesting aside to the rat study with respect to the development of metastasized prostate cancer was the realization that the rat research was not complete until the rodents' diets were changed to more closely approximate that of humans; that means their low-fat vegan diet was upped to more closely resemble the fat-rich American diet. With that change, the combined impact of the genes PTEN and PML was realized.)

The experts at Prostate Cancer UK take a somewhat more studied approach to the subject of prostate cancer and diet. They wrote:

A healthy diet and regular physical activity are important for general health and can help you stay a healthy weight. This may be particularly important if you've been diagnosed with prostate cancer, as there is strong evidence that being overweight or obese increases the risk of getting prostate cancer that's aggressive (more likely to spread) or advanced (cancer that has spread outside the prostate).

A healthy lifestyle can also help manage many of the side effects of treatments for prostate cancer.

We don't recommend any set diet or exercise programme. Instead, we suggest ways to improve your overall health, including some changes that might help with your prostate cancer.[9]

The consensus suggests that men living in the Mediterranean region and those living in Japan experience fewer incidence of prostate cancer than men in northern Europe and the United States. One reason could be that the diets in the Mediterranean and Japan are high in vegetables and healthful herbs, fish, and soy foods, which tend to replace red meats and dairy products. Those diets also favor whole grains over refined grains and foods made with flour and sugar. Both diets also contain a good dose of fiber.

While the actual diets of those two parts of the world differ in many ways, they have common characteristics that are distinguished by their cancer-fighting properties. Mediterranean cuisine tends to be characterized by tomato products, which as we have noted are known to be good sources of cancer-fighting Lycopene, as well as the antioxidants found in extra virgin olive oil. Rosemary and oregano, common in foods from the Mediterranean region, also have cancer-fighting properties.

The Japanese diet, however, is quite different. In a Cancer Science report about a "case-control study of diet and prostate cancer in Japan," the authors said that the "results provide support [for] the hypothesis that the traditional Japanese diet, which is rich in soybean products and fish, might be protective against prostate cancer."[10]

Harvard researchers have arrived at essentially the same conclusion. Researchers at the university reported that the incidence of prostate cancer—especially aggressive prostate cancer—is higher in countries where men eat a typical "Western" diet, one that contains a large amount of meat as opposed to the plant-based foods that are characteristic of Asian diets.

These studies have shown this correlation, unfortunately, those studies were not designed to prove cause-and-effect. Therefore, "definitive answers about prostate cancer and diet aren't yet in—although researchers are actively studying this topic," Harvard reports.

Even so, *Johns Hopkins' Discovery* has reported on extensive research by passionate nutritionist Dr. Bill Nelson and concluded: "Charred Food Bad, Veggies Good for the Prostate."[11] According to Nelson, the "bottom line" is: What should you be eating or not eating to reduce your risk of prostate cancer? Eating plenty of fruits and vegetables and consuming less red meat are things we've already discussed, but other important ingredients of a healthy diet include:

- Vitamin E: "Although the evidence in favor of Vitamin E is not as strong as that supporting selenium, Nelson believes it looks promising."
- Lycopene: Lycopene has gotten a lot of promising publicity, but whether lycopene can prevent prostate cancer "has not yet been proven," cautions Dr. Nelson. Research studies, which take years to complete, will eventually tell the story.
- Green tea: The big question remains: is consumption of large amounts of green tea the reason that people in Asia get less prostate cancer? Nelson asks, although the Asian diet is quite different from the Western diet. Is it harmful? Probably not. Will it work? Obviously, the Chinese drink a lot of it; there is stuff in there that's biologically active. Beyond that, it's anybody's guess.
- Soy: Soy contains cancer-fighting products called isoflavones, including one called genistein, which has been purported to fight cancer cells. Soy is, indeed, a staple of the Asian diet, but even this is complicated: "If you are deriving a lot of your protein nutrition from soy products, that means you probably aren't deriving it from other sources," such as red meat. Which brings us to the "sins of omission and sins of commission" argument. Is soy good for us because of some key ingredient or does it prevent cancer because we're eating it instead of red meat?
- Sulforaphane: Healthline describes sulforaphane as a natural plant compound found in many cruciferous vegetables (broccoli, cabbage, cauliflower, and kale)."[12] Sulforaphane seems to protect against several cancers by turning up the body's production of protective enzymes, but it's not yet clear, says Nelson, whether prostate cancer is one of them.
- Coffee: In the "Science of Living Well," the Prostate Cancer Foundation notes that coffee was once associated with poor health. It turns out, however, that a 2018 study "revealed that what was initially thought to be a link between coffee and cancer turned out to be a link between smoking and cancer" since many people smoked when they drank coffee.[13] However, the PCF says that "two studies have found that the antioxidants in coffee may reduce the risk

of prostate cancer." Who knew, or as they say, "what is old is new again."

- Red grapes: Several sources cite red grapes as having positive anti-cancer properties—besides, the seedless ones are fun to eat. Dr. Stefano Tiziani, assistant professor at the Department of Nutritional Sciences and Dell Pediatric Research Institute at the University of Texas at Austin, says that the nutrients in red grapes "have potential anti-cancer properties and are readily available." Unfortunately, he adds, "We only need to increase concentration beyond levels found in a healthy diet for an effect on prostate cancer cells."[14] We say, "eat 'em, anyway."

- Mushrooms: The *International Journal of Cancer* "found an inverse relationship between mushroom consumption and the development of prostate cancer among middle-aged and elderly Japanese men, suggesting that regular mushroom intake might help prevent prostate cancer."[15] However, no mention was made of the nationality's lower statistical rate of prostate cancer. There were two studies involving 36,499 men ages forty to seventy-nine that ran for 13.2 years. They suggested up to a "17% lower risk" of prostate cancer among the heavy consumers of mushrooms, but since the studies did not report information on the specific species of mushrooms—and there are thousands—that were consumed, the results remain uncertain. *Science Daily* reported that the lead author, Shu Zhang, PhD at the Tohoku University of Public Health in Japan, admitted, "The mechanism of the beneficial effects of mushroom on prostate cancer remain uncertain." Men might want to question the veracity of this information since the website Mushroom-Appreciation.com says, "There are over 10,000 types of mushrooms," which it admits is likely a modest total estimate of the mushroom universe.[16]

And finally, a really "bad guy" is charred meat. We create carcinogens, or cancer-causing agents, with every pork chop, steak, or hamburger we grill or fry. "Cooking meat at high temperatures produces cancer-causing chemicals called heterocyclic amines (HCAs), particularly if it produces char marks," says Dr. Stephen Freedland, director of the Center for Integrated Research in Cancer and Lifestyle.[17] "Plus, when fat drips into the grill, the resulting flames can cover food with polyaromatic hydrocarbons (PAHs), another chemical linked to cancer."

In choosing your daily diet, *Web*MD recommends the following:[18]

Eat and drink less of these. . .

- Reduce overall calories!
- Avoid flax seed oil.
- Avoid high-calcium diets.
- Avoid high-dose zinc supplements.
- Avoid excess preserved, pickled. or salted foods.
- Avoid trans fatty acids that are found in margarines and fried and baked foods.
- Avoid oils high in polyunsaturated fats such as corn, canola, or soybean.
- Avoid cured meats, such as salami, bacon, luncheon meats, and hot dogs that contain nitrites.
- Avoid white vegetables, such as potatoes and rice as well as flour and sugar.
- Avoid saturated fats such as fatty meats, egg yolks, dairy products, coconut oil, palm oil, and cottonseed oil.
- Cut down on sugary commercial sodas, including diet sodas.
- Reduce animal fat, especially that from red meat and high-fat dairy products.
- Reduce the intake of calcium. Men with the highest intake of calcium (including supplements) had a 39 percent increased risk of prostate cancer.

Eat and drink more of these. . .

- Drink water, which can speed metabolism and flush cancer-causing substances.
- Drink green tea several times each week.
- Eat fresh cold-water fish at least two to three times a week. Salmon, sardines, mackerel, and trout contain alpha omega-3 fatty acids. These should be poached, baked, or grilled (not burned or charred). Avoid fried fish.

- Eat more cabbage, broccoli, cauliflower, and tomatoes and tomato products, which includes pizza sauce, tomato paste, and ketchup.
- Eat red grapes and drink red grape juice or red wine regularly.
- Significantly increase your green leafy vegetables, fresh herbs, nuts, berries, and seeds.
- Increase your vitamin C consumption with citrus, berries, spinach, cantaloupe, sweet peppers, and mango.
- Use olive oil, which is very healthy and rich in vitamin E and anti-oxidants. Avocado oil is also good.
- Take a multivitamin with B complex and folic acid daily.
- Take vitamin E, 50 to 100 IU of gamma and d-alpha (only with the approval of your doctor. Some recent studies have raised concerns over serious risks with vitamin E intake). Natural sources include nuts, seeds, olive oil, avocado oil, wheat germ, peas, and nonfat milk.
- Selenium is a very powerful antioxidant and the backbone molecule of your body's immune system. Most studies support a daily selenium supplement of 200 micrograms a day. Since it only costs about 7 cents a day and is not toxic at these levels, it is reasonable for all men to take selenium. Natural sources include Brazil nuts, fresh fish, grains, mushrooms, wheat germ, bran, whole wheat bread, oats, and brown rice.

*Web*MD recommendations regarding these foods echo those of Johns Hopkins University, Harvard University, and Hearst.

*Web*MD also concurs with the Mayo Clinic's statements on rules-of-the-road for men receiving prostate cancer treatment or wishing to prevent it. Their list follows:

1. Moderation is the key. Don't follow these or any guidelines to excess.
2. Exercise regularly; walking is best.
3. Limit your calorie intake. Eat what you need to get to the next meal, not the usual American style of eating, that is, as if you're never going to eat again.
4. Get sunshine daily, but in moderation.
5. Variety in the foods you eat is important.

6. Remember that supplements are supplements and not intended to replace an intelligent diet.

In addition, the Prostate Cancer Foundation notes that the existence of stress can have a negative impact on your body's ability to resist prostate cancer and its spread. The PCF reports that "Studies have found that stress can trigger a physical reaction that appears to contribute to and/or exacerbate conditions including asthma, arthritis, depression, cardiovascular disease, chronic pain, HIV/AIDS, stroke, obesity and certain types of cancers," including prostate cancer.

Therefore, the PCF says, "it is important to keep stress levels in check," and they suggest the following ways to achieve that:

- Accept your points of stress and don't become "stressed out" by them.
- Spend time with friends.
- Try yoga to connect the mind and body.
- Engage in nonsexual affection such as hugging.
- Laughter is good medicine.
- Pets alleviate stress-related blood pressure increases.
- Exercise! Work up a sweat.
- Crying provides a release and reduces stress.
- Sleep well, and long enough, at night.

DIETARY SUPPLEMENTS

Nutritional and herbal supplements—added to your daily diet and in connection with conventional medical treatment—have long been credited with helping fight prostate cancer. If you have prostate cancer, British researchers have scientifically proven that that some substances fight prostate cancer, including:

- Broccoli
- Turmeric [curcumin]
- Green tea, pomegranate, and pomegranate juice

Cambridge University Hospital oncologist Professor Robert Thomas and his team conducted a relatively small, six-month study among 203 adult men with prostate cancer. The men were split into two groups: one took a daily capsule containing the essence of pomegranate, turmeric, green tea, and broccoli. The second control group took a placebo. In this double-blind study, neither the doctors nor the participants knew who were taking the placebo capsules and who was not taking them. After six months, the researchers found that PSA levels were 63 percent lower among those taking capsules containing essence of pomegranate, turmeric, green tea, and broccoli compared to those in the placebo group.

The Mayo Cancer Center research, however, disputes the value of pomegranate juice. Mayo's Dr. Erik P. Castle wrote in May 2019, "Some early research suggested that drinking pomegranate juice slowed the progression of prostate cancer, but additional research failed to confirm those results."[19] He also wrote, "In some studies of men with recurrent prostate cancer and rising Prostate-Specific Antigen levels, researchers found that drinking pomegranate juice or taking pomegranate juice extract significantly slowed the rate at which PSA was rising (PSA doubling time). A longer PSA doubling time can indicate that the cancer may be progressing less rapidly."

Dr. Castle disagrees with "the placebo-controlled" British study that found value in consuming the pomegranate cocktail, so perhaps we can assign those positive results to the other ingredients: turmeric, green tea, and broccoli. As with so many things medical, there is little unanimity on many medical issues.

Another stand-alone supplement is turmeric. It is a commercially available nutritional supplement that is purported to treat some forms of prostate cancer, as well as other diseases. Its use is also controversial and yet proven to be effective. Memorial Sloan Kettering reports:

> Recent experiments suggest turmeric [the source of curcumin] may interfere with the activity of some chemotherapy drugs, so the question remains whether this spice is helpful or harmful during chemotherapy.

A paper published in *BioMed Central* (BMC) claims that "curcumin . . . is a promising chemo-preventive compound, that appears [to be an appropriate] non-toxic alternative for prostate cancer prevention, treatment or co-treatment." The paper explains, however, that "despite the fact that curcumin is well described in several cancer types for its anti-oxidant potential . . . nothing was published [until this paper] concerning prostate cancer."

The paper further notes that "several data pointed out that curcumin is able to suppress the proliferation of both androgen-dependent and androgen-independent prostate cancer cell line(s). . . . "This natural compound also promotes the [initiation] of prostate cancer cell death . . . and could be useful in combination with conventional treatment such as immunotherapy and radiotherapy," concluding that "curcumin may prevent the progression of prostate cancer . . . treat advanced prostate cancer."

So, if you plan to use turmeric, or curcumin, talk to your doctor first.

WHAT ABOUT SUGAR?

On a somewhat lighter note, MedicineNet.com provides a quick but interesting comparison of a number of common foods and the amount of sugar each contains.[20] While the study was designed to help those seeking to lose weight, it provides results that are, at best, amazing, troubling, and somewhat relevant to diet related to prostate cancer.

Grab a pencil and circle which (below) you believe has more sugar. The answers follow.

- Ketchup or Mustard
- Soft Drink or Bottled Apple Juice
- Dried Cranberries or Gummy Bears
- Boston Cream Doughnut or Mocha Frappuccino
- Raisin Bran or Blueberry Waffle
- Jarred Tomato Sauce or Strawberries
- Mayonnaise or Creamy Salad Dressing
- Canned Peaches or Chocolate Chip Cookies
- Caramel Corn or Prepackaged Cole Slaw
- Instant Oatmeal or Pancakes
- Candy Bar or Granola Bar

Here are the answers; the items with the greater amount of sugar are underlined and in bold.

- **<u>Ketchup 14g per tablespoon</u>** or Mustard 0.14g per tablespoon
- Soft drink 39g per 12 oz. serving or **<u>Apple juice 42g per 12 oz. serving</u>**
- **<u>Dried cranberries 60g per half cup</u>** or Gummy Bears 30g per half cup
- Boston cream doughnut 20g per 16 oz. or **<u>Mocha frappuccino 61g per 16 oz.</u>**
- **<u>Raisin bran 18g per cup</u>** or Blueberry waffle 3g per cup
- **<u>Jarred tomato sauce 16g per cup</u>** or Strawberries 5g per cup
- **<u>Mayonnaise 5g per 2 tablespoons</u>** or Creamy salad dressing 3–4g per 2 tablespoons
- **<u>Canned peaches 16g per half cup</u>** or Chocolate chip cookies 11g in 3 cookies
- Caramel corn 6–7g per half cup or **<u>Creamy cole slaw 13g per half cup</u>**
- **<u>Instant oatmeal 12+g per packet</u>** or 3 4-inch pancakes 5g
- **<u>Candy bar 27g per regular size bar</u>** or Granola bar ~13g per same size bar

IN OUR OPINION. . .

We agree with the many doctors who suggest that living a "healthy lifestyle" as described earlier in this chapter is an appropriate way to moderate your chances of developing this dreadful disease.

We find it particularly noteworthy that evidence shows that Southeast Asian men typically have low levels of prostate cancer while living in their homelands; however, when they relocate to the West, especially North America, their levels of prostate cancer rise considerably.

Compare the typical diet of an American male with that of an Asian and you will see that the American eats more fatty red (and often char-cooked) meat, eats fewer green vegetables, eats more starches like potatoes, and generally is overweight. Frankly, the statistics speak for themselves.

As for dietary supplements, and other novel cocktails of juices, those seem to be largely untested, and the impacts for good or ill are largely undetermined.

Our recommendation is disgustingly plain: All things in moderation.

- *Eat moderately of largely natural foods.*
- *Let your foods lean to the colorful side.*
- *Eat little meat, and no charred meat.*
- *Exercise sufficiently.*
- *Maintain a healthy weight.*
- *Reduce the complexity and anxiety in your life.*

25

How Does Prostate Cancer Spread?

Prostate cancer, regardless of what part of the body it moves to, is still prostate cancer. That is the case whether it travels to your pelvis or to your lungs; it is still prostate cancer. In a sense, you can never really get rid of it even though you may think that you have. Therefore, it is important to understand how prostate cancer spreads, and what you can do to deal with it. That's what this chapter is all about, understanding the demon and how to fight it.

Cancer is considered such a serious disease because of its ability to spread from its point of origin in the prostate into otherwise normal tissue in other parts of the body. Cancer can also spread near its point of origin to nearby lymph nodes. When it establishes itself in other parts of the body away from its point of origin, it's called metastatic prostate cancer. This process of cancer cells spreading to distant parts of the body is called metastasis.

This spreading of the cancer cells happens when a few of the cells break away from the main tumor and travel to the blood stream or the lymph system. Once there, they move through your body until they stop in tiny blood vessels called capillaries. They then multiply and grow new blood vessels to bring nutrients to the new tumor. Prostate cancer prefers to grow in tissue areas such as lymph nodes or in the bones.

While breakaway cancer cells form new tumors, many others don't survive in the bloodstream. Some die at the site of the new tissue, while others may lie inactive for years or never become active."[1]

According to the American Cancer Society (ACS), the newly developed tumors need not be exactly like the ones from which they originated, which might make them harder to treat.

If your prostate cancer spreads to another part of your body, say to a bone, it is not bone cancer; it is still "prostate cancer," but it's called "prostate cancer in the bone." These metastatic prostate cancer cells, regardless of where they reside, usually have features in common with the cells at their point of origin; that is how doctors can determine where they came from. (Sometimes, however, metastatic cancer is diagnosed when the point of origin is unknown, and this is called a CUP, Carcinoma of Unknown Primary.)

The ACS very clearly explains how cancer spreads:

> Where a cancer starts is linked to where it will spread. Most cancer cells that break free from the original tumor are carried in the blood or lymph system until they get trapped in the next "downstream" organ or set of lymph nodes. Once the cells are there, they can start to grow and form new tumors.
>
> This explains why breast cancer often spreads to underarm lymph nodes, but rarely to lymph nodes in the groin.
>
> Likewise, there are many cancers that commonly spread to the lungs. This is because the heart pumps blood from the rest of the body through the lungs' blood vessels before sending it elsewhere.

Although cancer can spread to any bone in the body, it usually spreads to a bone nearby, and is most often found in bones near the center of the body. "The spine is the most common site" according to the ACS. Other common sites are the hip, pelvis, upper leg bone, upper arm bone, ribs, and the skull. Additionally, the National Cancer Institute says that prostate cancer can also metastasize to the adrenal gland, liver, and lungs.[2]

> Once cancer has spread to the bones or to other parts of the body it's rarely able to be cured. Still, it often can be treated to shrink, stop, or slow its growth. Even if a cure is no longer possible, treating the cancer may be able to help you live longer and feel better.

Unfortunately, metastatic cancer does not always cause symptoms. When symptoms do occur, their nature and frequency will depend on the size and location of the metastatic tumors. Some common signs of metastatic cancer include the following:

- Pain and fractures when cancer has spread to the bone.

- Headache, seizures, or dizziness when cancer has spread to the brain.
- Shortness of breath when cancer has spread to the lungs.
- Jaundice or swelling in the belly when cancer has spread to the liver.

Healthline reports that about 80 percent of the time, prostate cancer metastasizes to bones, such as the hip, spine, or pelvis.[3] Symptoms of bone metastases of prostate cancer include the following:

- Bloody urine or semen
- Erectile dysfunction
- Painful ejaculation
- Swelling in pelvic area or legs
- Fatigue
- Unexplained weight loss

While no cure for metastatic prostate cancer is currently available, new therapies that extend life are in clinical trials and coming to market regularly. Different treatments affect men differently, and your doctor or personal decision assistant, or PDA, will be able to discuss your long-term outlook with you. This can be helpful when making plans for the future.

IN OUR OPINION. . .

Perhaps it is appropriate that we end this book with the section on metastases of prostate cancer. From our first pages, we have taken you from the day you first heard the fateful words of your internist, "You may have prostate cancer," through the many phases of the disease, and now to the last and most difficult aspect of it, the metastases.

Hopefully, we have answered many of your questions, though we are certain that you have many more, and many that are specific to your own condition. That's where your oncology team and PDA come in. They should be able to provide you with the information you need, though it may not be the information you want.

As we end this book, we are comforted in the belief that new treatments—one of us is in a clinical trial as we write these words—coming online almost daily. This is an indication that prostate cancer is finally getting the attention it deserves. It is a dreadful disease, one that robs men of much of what makes them a man, and it must be stopped.

Good luck with your fight!

Resources for Information and Treatment

PROSTATE CANCER WEBSITES

Below are numerous potentially useful prostate cancer websites. This is not intended to be an exhaustive list, but we think these sites will be useful for prostate cancer patients and those close to them.

You may have to search "prostate cancer" at some of these sites.

- American Cancer Society: https://www.cancer.org
- Cleveland Clinic: https://my.clevelandclinic.org
- Cornell University Hospital: https://weill.cornell.edu
- Dana-Farber Cancer Institute: http://www.dfbwcc.org
- Healing Well: https://www.healingwell.com/prostatecancer/
- Early Prostate Cancer: http://www.medicinenet.com/
- His Prostate Cancer: http://www.hisprostatecancer.com
- Johns Hopkins University Hospital: https://www.jhu.edu
- Know Your Prostate Plan: https://www.knowyourprostateplan.com/
- Massachusetts General Hospital: https://www.massgeneral.org
- Massachusetts General-Brigham: https://www.brighamandwomens.org
- Mayo Clinic: https://www.mayoclinic.org
- My Prostate Cancer Roadmap: https://www.myprostatecancerroadmap.com/
- Presbyterian Hospital–Columbia: https://www.nyp.org
- Prostate Cancer FAQs: http://prostatecancer911.com
- Prostate Cancer Foundation: https://www.pcf.org

- Cancer Treatment Centers of America: http://www.cancercenter.com/prostate-cancer/
- Top Prostate Cancer Questions: http://www.hopkinsmedicine.org
- University of California Los Angeles Medical Center: https://www.uclahealth.org/reagan/
- University of California San Francisco: https://www.ucsf.edu
- University of Rochester Medical Center: https://www.urmc.rochester.edu
- *Web*MD: http://www.webmd.com

TOP 20 HOSPITALS AS RANKED BY
U.S. NEWS AND *NEWSWEEK*

U.S. News began evaluating hospitals three decades ago and has periodically revamped the way it measures them to improve their decisions.

Newsweek has ranked hospitals for the two years and takes a global approach, as opposed to the domestic view used at *U.S. News*. The full lists are available at: *U.S. News* and *Newsweek*.

U.S. News's Top 20 Hospitals in the United States

1. Mayo Clinic, Rochester, Minnesota
2. Cleveland Clinic, Ohio
3. Johns Hopkins Hospital, Baltimore
4. (tie) Presbyterian Hospital–Columbia and Cornell, New York City
5. (tie) University of California Medical Center, Los Angeles
6. Massachusetts General Hospital, Boston
7. Cedars-Sinai Medical Center, San Francisco
8. University of California Medical Center, San Francisco
9. New York University Langone Hospitals, New York City
10. Northwestern Memorial Hospital, Chicago
11. University of Michigan Hospitals, Ann Arbor
12. Brigham and Women's Hospital, Boston
13. Stanford Health Care–Stanford Hospital, Palo Alto
14. Mount Sinai Hospital, New York City
15. Hospitals of the University of Pennsylvania–Penn Presbyterian

16. Mayo Clinic–Phoenix
17. Rush University Medical Center, Chicago
18. (tie) Barnes-Jewish Hospital, Saint Louis
19. (tie) Keck Hospital of University of Southern California, Los Angeles
20. Houston Methodist Hospital, Texas

Newsweek's Top 20 Hospitals in the World

1. Mayo Clinic, Rochester
2. Cleveland Clinic, Ohio
3. Massachusetts General Hospital, Boston
4. Toronto General Hospital
5. Charité–Universitätsmedizin, Berlin
6. Johns Hopkins University Hospital, Baltimore
7. Universitätsspital, Zürich
8. Singapore General Hospital
9. Sheba Medical Center, Ramat Gan, Israel
10. Karolinska Universitetssjukhuset, Solna, Sweden
11. Aarhus Universitetshospital, Aarhus, Denmark
12. Hôpital Universitaire Pitié Salpêtrière, Paris
13. Centre Hospitalier Universitaire Vaudois, Lausanne
14. Universitätsklinikum, Heidelberg
15. University of Michigan Hospitals, Ann Arbor
16. St. Luke's International Hospital, Tokyo
17. Brigham and Women's Hospital, Boston
18. The University of Tokyo Hospital, Tokyo
19. Rigshospitalet–København, Copenhagen
20. UMC Utrecht, Utrecht, Netherlands

NATIONAL CANCER INSTITUTE– DESIGNATED CANCER CENTERS

The National Cancer Institute has designated more than sixty facilities as either "Cancer Centers" or "Comprehensive Cancer Centers," which are listed next. The following link will take you to its home page:

https://www.cancer.net/navigating-cancer-care/cancer-basics/cancer -care-team/find-nci-designated-cancer-center. The descriptions below are also from its website.

"**Cancer Centers.** Cancer Centers integrate research activities across three major areas: laboratory research, clinical research, and population-based research. Many of these centers also provide care and services for cancer patients."

"**Comprehensive Cancer Centers**. In addition to the same activities conducted by Cancer Centers, Comprehensive Cancer Centers also have extensive community outreach and education programs."

"**Cooperative Groups**. The NCI Cooperative Groups are large networks of researchers, doctors, and health-care professionals at public and private institutions that conduct multi-center, large-scale, phase III cancer clinical trials across the country."

Following is a list of Cancer Centers and Comprehensive Cancer Centers. They are listed alphabetically.

Abramson Comprehensive Cancer Center
3400 Spruce Street
Philadelphia, PA 19104
215-615-5858
http://www.penncancer.org/

Albert Einstein Cancer Center
Albert Einstein College of Medicine
1300 Morris Park Avenue
Bronx, NY 10461
718-862-8840
http://www.einstein.yu.edu/centers/cancer/

Cancer Therapy and Research Center
University of Texas Health Science Center
7979 Wurzbach Road
San Antonio, TX 78229
210-450-1000
http://www.ctrc.net

Case Comprehensive Cancer Center
11100 Euclid Avenue
Cleveland, OH 44106
216-844-8797
http://cancer.case.edu

Chao Family Comprehensive Cancer Center
101 The City Drive
Building 56, Rt. 81, Room 216L
Orange, CA 92868
714-456-8000
http://www.cancer.uci.edu

City of Hope Comprehensive Cancer Center
1500 East Duarte Road
Duarte, CA 91010
626-256-4673
https://www.cityofhope.org/homepage

Columbia University Irving Comprehensive Cancer Center
1130 St. Nicholas Avenue, Room 201
New York, NY 10032
212-305-2500

Duncan Comprehensive Cancer Center
Baylor College of Medicine
One Baylor Place
MS: BCM305
Houston, TX 77030
713-798-1354
https://www.bcm.edu/centers/cancer-center

Dana-Farber/Harvard Comprehensive Cancer Center
450 Brookline Avenue
Boston, MA 02215
617-632-3000
http://www.dfhcc.harvard.edu/

Duke Comprehensive Cancer Center
Duke University Medical Center
Box 2714
2424 Erwin Road
Durham, NC 27710
888-275-3853
http://cancer.duke.edu

Fox Chase Comprehensive Cancer Center
333 Cottman Avenue
Philadelphia, PA 19111-2497
215-728-2570
http://www.fccc.edu

Fred and Pamela Buffett Cancer Center
University of Nebraska Medical Center
505 South 45th Street, Omaha, NE 68106
402-559-6500
https://www.unmc.edu/cancercenter/

Fred Hutchinson Comprehensive Cancer Center
P.O. Box 19024, D1-060
Seattle, WA 98109
206-288-1024
http://www.cancerconsortium.org/en.html

Georgetown Lombardi Comprehensive Cancer Center
3970 Reservoir Rd., NW
Washington, DC 20007
202-444-2223
http://lombardi.georgetown.edu

Holden Comprehensive Cancer Center
200 Hawkins Drive 5970Z JPP
Iowa City, IA 52242
319-356-4200
https://uihc.org/primary-and-specialty-care/holden-comprehensive
    -cancer-center

Hollings Cancer Center
Medical University of South Carolina
86 Jonathan Lucas Street
Charleston, SC 29425
843-792-0700
http://hcc.musc.edu/

Huntsman Institute Comprehensive Cancer Center
2000 Circle of Hope
Salt Lake City, UT 84112
877-585-0303
http://www.huntsmancancer.org

Indiana University Simon Cancer Center
535 Barnhill Drive
Indianapolis, IN 46202
317-944-5000
http://cancer.iu.edu

Karmanos Comprehensive Cancer Center
Wayne State University School of Medicine
4100 John R. Street
Detroit, MI 48201
800-527-6266
http://www.karmanos.org

Kimmel Cancer Center at Thomas Jefferson University
233 South 10th Street
Philadelphia, PA 19107
215-503-4500
http://www.kimmelcancercenter.org

Kimmel Comprehensive Cancer Center
401 North Broadway
Baltimore, MD 21231
410-955-8964
https://www.cancer.gov/research/nci-role/cancer-centers/find/hopkins
    kimmel

Knight Institute Comprehensive Cancer Center
Oregon Health and Science University
3181 South West Sam Jackson Park Road
Portland, OR 97239
503-494-1617
http://www.ohsu.edu/health/cancer/index.html

Lurie Comprehensive Cancer Center
303 East Superior Street
Chicago, IL 60611
312-695-0990
http://www.cancer.northwestern.edu

Markey Cancer Center
CC140 Roach Building
800 Rose Street
Lexington, KY 40536-0096
859-257-4500
https://ukhealthcare.uky.edu/markey-cancer-center

Maryland Greenebaum Comprehensive Cancer Center
22 South Greene Street
Baltimore, MD 21201
410-328-7904
https://www.umms.org/umgccc

Masonic Comprehensive Cancer Center
420 Delaware Street, South East
Minneapolis, MN 55455
612-672-7422
http://www.cancer.umn.edu/

Massey Cancer Center
P.O. Box 980037
401 College Street
Richmond, VA 23298
804-828-5116
http://www.massey.vcu.edu

Mayo Clinic Comprehensive Cancer Center
200 First Street South West
Rochester, MN 55905
507-284-2511
https://www.mayoclinic.org/departments-centers/mayo-clinic-cancer
-center

Mays Cancer Center
UT Health Science Center
7979 Wurzbach Road
Urschel Tower, Room U627
San Antonio, TX 78229
210-450-1000
https://www.uthscsa.edu/patient-care/cancer-center/

Memorial Sloan Kettering Comprehensive Cancer Center
1275 York Ave.
New York, NY 10065
212-639-2000
http://www.mskcc.org

Moffitt Cancer Center
12902 Magnolia Drive
MCC-CEO
Tampa, FL 33612
813-745-4673
http://www.moffitt.org

New York University Perlmutter Cancer Center
550 First Avenue
1201 Smilow Building
New York, NY
212-731-6000
https://nyulangone.org/locations/perlmutter-cancer-center

Norris Cotton Comprehensive Cancer Center
Dartmouth-Hitchcock Medical Center
One Medical Center Drive
Lebanon, NH 03756
603-653-9000
http://www.cancer.dartmouth.edu

Ohio State University Comprehensive Cancer Center
James Cancer Hospital and Solove Research Institute
650 Ackerman Road
Columbus, OH 43202
614-293-5066
https://cancer.osu.edu/

O'Neal Comprehensive Cancer Center
University of Alabama at Birmingham
Birmingham, AL 35294
205-975-8222
https://www.uab.edu/onealcancercenter/

Roswell Park Comprehensive Cancer
Elm & Carlton Streets
Buffalo, NY 14263
716-845-2300
http://www.roswellpark.org

Rutgers Comprehensive Cancer Center
195 Little Albany St.
New Brunswick, NJ 08903
732-235-2465
http://www.cinj.org

St. Jude Children's Research Hospital Comprehensive Cancer Center
262 Danny Thomas Place
Memphis, TN 38105
866-278-5833
https://www.stjude.org/

Simmons Comprehensive Cancer Center
Southwestern Medical Center
2201 Inwood Road
Dallas, TX 75390
214-645-4673
http://www.utswmedicine.org/conditions-specialties/cancer/

Siteman Comprehensive Cancer Center
Washington University School of Medicine
Campus Box 8109
St. Louis, MO 63110
314-747-7222
http://www.siteman.wustl.edu

Stanford Comprehensive Cancer Center
Lorry Lokey Stem Cell Building
265 Campus Drive, Suite G2103
Stanford, CA 94305
650-498-6000
http://cancer.stanford.edu

Stephenson Cancer Center
800 Northeast 10th Street
Oklahoma City, OK 73104
405-271-1112
http://stephensoncancercenter.org/

Sylvester Comprehensive Cancer Center
UM Miller School of Medicine
1475 NW 12th Avenue
Miami, FL 33136
305-243-1000
https://umiamihealth.org/sylvester-comprehensive-cancer-center

Tisch Cancer Institute at Mount Sinai
One Gustave L. Levy Place
PO Box 1128
Icahn Building, 1st Floor
New York, NY 10029
212-659-5600
http://icahn.mssm.edu/research/tisch

University of Arizona Comprehensive Cancer Center
1515 North Campbell Avenue
Tucson, AZ 85724-5024
800-524-5928
http://www.azcc.arizona.edu

University of California Davis Comprehensive Cancer Center
4501 X Street, Suite 3003
Sacramento, CA 95817
916-703-5210
http://ucdmc.ucdavis.edu/cancer/

University of California Los Angeles Jonsson Comprehensive Cancer
    Center
8-684 Factor Building,
10833 Le Conte Avenue
Los Angeles, CA 90095-1781
888-662-8252
http://www.cancer.ucla.edu

University of California San Diego Moores Comprehensive Cancer
3855 Health Sciences Drive
La Jolla, CA 92093
858-822-6100
https://health.ucsd.edu/specialties/cancer/Pages/default.aspx

University of California San Francisco Helen Diller Family Comprehensive Cancer Center
1450 3rd Street, Box 0128
San Francisco, CA 94115
888-689-8273
http://cancer.ucsf.edu/

University of Chicago Comprehensive Cancer Center
5841 South Maryland Avenue MC1140
Chicago, IL 60637
Pediatric: 773-702-6808
Adult: 855-702-8222
https://cancer.uchicago.edu/

University of Colorado Comprehensive Cancer
13001 East 17th Place
Aurora, CO 80045
Adult: 720-848-0300
Pediatric: 720-777-6688
http://www.uccc.info

University of Hawaii Cancer Center
701 Ilalo Street
Suite 600
Honolulu, HI 96813
808-586-3010
http://www.uhcancercenter.org/

University of Kansas Cancer Center
3901 Rainbow Boulevard
Kansas City, KS 66160
913-588-1227
https://www.kucancercenter.org/

University of Michigan Comprehensive Cancer Center
1500 East Medical Center Dr.
Ann Arbor, MI 48109-0944
800-865-1125
http://www.cancer.med.umich.edu

University of New Mexico Comprehensive Cancer
1201 Camino de Salud, North East
Albuquerque, NM 87131
505-272-4946
http://cancer.unm.edu

University of North Carolina Lineberger Comprehensive Cancer
    Center
450 West Drive, CB 7295
Chapel Hill, NC 27599
919-966-3036
http://www.unclineberger.org

University of Pittsburgh Medical Center Hillman Cancer Center
5150 Centre Avenue
Pittsburgh, PA 15232
412-647-2811
http://upci.upmc.edu/index.cfm

University of Southern California Norris Comprehensive Cancer
    Center
1441 Eastlake Avenue
Los Angeles, CA 90089
323-865-3000
http://uscnorriscancer.usc.edu/

University of Texas MD Anderson Comprehensive Cancer
1515 Holcombe Blvd., Unit 91
Houston, TX 77030
713-792-6161
http://www.mdanderson.org

University of Virginia Cancer Center
6171 West Complex
Charlottesville, VA 22908
434-924-3627
https://cancer.uvahealth.com/

Vanderbilt Ingram Comprehensive Cancer Center
691 Preston Research Building
Nashville, TN 37232
615-936-8422
http://www.vicc.org

Wake Forest Baptist Comprehensive Cancer Center
Medical Center Boulevard
Winston-Salem, NC 27157
336-716-7971
http://www.wakehealth.edu/Comprehensive-Cancer-Center/

Winship Comprehensive Cancer Center
1365C Clifton Road
Atlanta, GA 30322
404-778-1900
http://cancer.emory.edu/

Wisconsin Carbone Comprehensive Cancer Center
1111 Highland Avenue, Rm. 7057
Madison, WI 53792
608-263-8600
https://www.uwhealth.org/uw-carbone-cancer-center/47424

Yale Comprehensive Cancer Center
PO Box 208028
New Haven, CT 06520-8028
877-925-3637
http://yalecancercenter.org/

Bibliography

A

Advanced Urological Care P.C. "Penile Injection Therapy." Accessed September 23, 2020. https://www.urologicalcare.com/erectile-dysfunction/penile-injection-therapy/.

Aetna Policy Bulletin. "Prostate Cancer Screening." Number 0521. April 26, 2019. http://www.aetna.com/cpb/medical/data/500_599/0521.html.

Alemozaffar, Mehrdad, Meredith M. Regan, Matthew R. Cooperberg et al. "Prediction of Erectile Function Following Treatment for Prostate Cancer." *Journal of the American Medical Association*, September 21, 2011. https://jamanetwork.com/journals/jama/fullarticle/1104401.

American Cancer Society. "Can Prostate Cancer Be Prevented?" Accessed July 15, 2020. https://www.cancer.org/cancer/prostate-cancer/early-detection/prevention.html.

American Cancer Society. "Cancer Statistics." Accessed July 2020. https://cancerstatisticscenter.cancer.org/?_ga=2.246550727.255157878.1594064649-1647637386.1594064649#!/.

American Cancer Society. "Cancer Statistics, 2017." January 5, 2017. https://acsjournals.onlinelibrary.wiley.com/doi/full/10.3322/caac.21387.

American Cancer Society. "Hormone Therapy for Prostate Cancer." Accessed April 21, 2019. https://www.cancer.org/cancer/prostate-cancer/treating/hormone-therapy.html.

American Cancer Society. "Insurance Coverage for Prostate Cancer Screening." Accessed August 1, 2019. https://www.cancer.org/cancer/prostate-cancer/early-detection/insurance-coverage.html.

American Cancer Society. "Key Statistics for Prostate Cancer." August 1, 2019. https://www.cancer.org/cancer/prostate-cancer/about/key-statistics.html.

American Cancer Society. "Prostate Cancer Risk Factors, Race/ethnicity." Accessed September 23, 2020. https://www.cancer.org/cancer/prostate-cancer/early-detection/risk-factors-for-prostate-cancer.html.

American Cancer Society. "Prostate Cancer Symptoms." Accessed July 11, 2020. https://www.webmd.com/prostate-cancer/guide/understanding-prostate-cancer-symptoms.

American Cancer Society. "Risk of Prostate Cancer." Accessed August 12, 2020. https://www.cancer.org/cancer/prostate-cancer/about/key-statistics.html.

American Cancer Society. "Signs and Symptoms of Prostate Cancer." Accessed August 1, 2019. https://www.cancer.org/cancer/prostate-cancer/detection-diagnosis-staging/signs-symptoms.html.

American Cancer Society. "Survival Rates for Prostate Cancer." Accessed July 2020. https://www.cancer.org/cancer/prostate-cancer/detection-diagnosis-staging/survival-rates.html.

American Cancer Society. "Tests for Prostate Cancer, Lymph Node Biopsy." Accessed September 23, 2020. https://www.cancer.org/cancer/prostate-cancer/detection-diagnosis-staging/how-diagnosed.html.

American Cancer Society. "Tests to Diagnose and Stage Prostate Cancer." Accessed September 10, 2020. https://www.cancer.org/cancer/prostate-cancer/detection-diagnosis-staging/how-diagnosed.html.

American Cancer Society. "Treating Prostate Cancer That Doesn't Go Away or Comes Back After Treatment." Accessed July 13, 2020. https://www.cancer.org/cancer/prostate-cancer/treating/recurrence.html.

American Family Physician. "Prostate Cancer Screening." October 15, 2015. https://www.aafp.org/afp/2015/1015/p683.html.

American Journal of Managed Care. "Management of Biochemically Recurrent Prostate Cancer Following Local Therapy." January 8, 2015. https://www.ajmc.com/journals/supplement/2014/ace021_dec14_prostate_ce/ace021_dec14_prostatece_kolodziej.

American Urological Association. "Early Detection of Prostate Cancer." Published 2013, Confirmed 2018. https://www.auanet.org/guidelines/prostate-cancer-early-detection-guideline.

Annals of Family Medicine. "National Evidence on the Use of Shared Decision Making in Prostate-Specific Antigen Screening." July 2013. https://www.ncbi.nlm.nih.gov/pmc/articles/PMC3704490/.

ASCO Post. "Psychosocial Case Is a Critical Component of Value-based Ocology." May 10, 2019. https://www.ascopost.com/issues/may-10-2019/psychosocial-care-is-a-critical-component-of-value-based-oncology.

B

Bankhead, Charles. "15 Percent of Men Regret Prostate Cancer Treatment Choices Years Later, Study Finds." *STAT*, July 12, 2017. https://www.stat news.com/2017/07/12/prostate-cancer-treatment-regret/.

Bapat, Ashwini C. "At Life's End, The Gift of Intimacy." WBUR-FM, May 14, 2019. https://www.wbur.org/cognoscenti/2019/05/14/palliative-care-dying -ashwini-bapat.

Basch E., K. Autio, C. J. Ryan et al. "Abiraterone Acetate Plus Prednisone Versus Prednisone Alone in Chemotherapy-naive Men with Metastatic Castration-resistant Prostate Cancer: Patient-reported Outcome Results of a Randomised Phase 3 Trial." *The Lancet Oncology*, September 25, 2013. https://www.the lancet.com/journals/lanonc/article/PIIS1470-2045(13)70424-8/fulltext.

Beth Israel Deaconess Medical Center. "Prostate Cancer Treatment by Stage." Accessed July 13, 2020. https://www.bidmc.org/centers-and-departments/ cancer-center/cancer-center-programs-and-services/prostate-cancer-center/ prostate-cancer-treatment-options.

Brigham Health Hub. "Prostate Cancer Screening: Who Recommends PSA Testing." Accessed July 10, 2019. https://brighamhealthhub.org/prevention/ prostate-cancer-screening-who-recommends-psa-testing.

British Association of Urological Surgeons. "Mortality Results from the Göteborg Randomized Population-based Prostate-Cancer Screening Trial." March 10, 2015. https://www.baus.org.uk/professionals/baus_business/ publications/21/prostate_cancer_screening.

British Journal of Urological Surgeons. "Prostate Cancer Screening." March 10, 2015. https://www.baus.org.uk/professionals/baus_business/ publications/21/prostate_cancer_screening.

Brownstein, Joseph. "Prostate Cancer Diagnosis May Bring Suicide, Heart Risks." ABC News, December 15, 2009. https://abcnews.go.com/Health/ ProstateCancerNews/prostate-cancer-diagnosis-brings-suicide-heart-risk/ story?id=9333628.

C

Canadian Task Force on Preventive Health Care. "Prostate Cancer—1000-person Tool." Accessed July 12, 2020. https://canadiantaskforce.ca/ tools-resources/prostate-cancer-harms-and-benefits/.

Cancer Research UK. "Screening." May 31, 2020. http://www.cancerresearchuk .org/about-cancer/prostate-cancer/getting-diagnosed/screening.

Cancer Treatment Centers of America. "Lymph Nodes." Accessed September 21, 2020. https://www.cancercenter.com/lymph-nodes.

Canfield, Steven E. "Annual Screening for Prostate Cancer Did Not Reduce Mortality from Prostate Cancer." *Annals of Internal Medicine*, June 16, 2009. http://annals.org/aim/article-abstract/744408/annual-screening -prostate-cancer-did-reduce-mortality-from-prostate-cancer.

Cedars Sinai. "Healthy Grilling: Reducing the Risk of Cancer." July 30, 2018. https://www.cedars-sinai.org/blog/grilling-cancer-risk.html.

Centers for Disease Control and Prevention. "HPV and Men Fact Sheet." December 28, 2016. https://www.cdc.gov/std/hpv/stdfact-hpv-and-men.htm.

Centers for Disease Control and Prevention. "Should I Get Screened for Prostate Cancer?" July 31, 2019. https://www.cdc.gov/cancer/prostate/ basic_info/get-screened.htm.

Chesler, Andrew. "The Importance of Identifying Anxiety and Depression in Men with Prostate Cancer." *Oncology Nursing News*, September 13, 2018. https://www.oncnursingnews.com/contributor/cancer-care/2018/09/the-imp ortance-of-identifying-anxiety-and-depression-in-men-with-prostate-cancer.

CIGNA. "Health Insurance." December 17, 2019. https://www.cigna.com/ individuals-families/health-wellness/hw/medical-topics/prostate-cancer -treatment-ncicdr0000062910.

Cleveland Clinic. "Laparoscopic Prostatectomy." Accessed September 21, 2020. https://my.clevelandclinic.org/health/treatments/17160-laparoscopic -prostatectomy.

Cleveland Clinic. "Prostate Cancer: Urinary Incontinence After Surgery: Procedure Details." June 2019. https://my.clevelandclinic.org/health/ treatments/8096-prostate-cancer-urinary-incontinence-after-surgery/proce dure-details.

Cleveland Clinic. "What Is the Prostate's Role in Urination?" Accessed July 13, 2020. https://my.clevelandclinic.org/health/treatments/8096-pros tate-cancer-urinary-incontinence-after-surgery.

Cochran.org. "About-us." Accessed July 13, 2020. http://www.cochrane.org/ about-us.

Columbia University Irving Medical Center. "Prostate Cancer Cryo-surgery Treatment." Accessed July 13, 2020. http://columbiaurology .org/adult-urology/urologic-oncology/prostate-cancer/prostate-cancer -cryosurgery-treatment.

Consult QD. "Metacure Trial: Can We Cure More Oligometastatic Prostate Cancer?" January 13, 2020. https://consultqd.clevelandclinic.org/ metacure-trial-can-we-cure-more-oligometastatic-prostate-cancer/.

D

Daley, Jim. "Prostate Cancer: Surgical Castration Linked to Fewer Adverse Events Than Chemical Castration." Cancer Therapy Advisor. January 21,

2016. https://www.cancertherapyadvisor.com/prostate-cancer/prostate
-cancer-surgery-castration-fewer-adverse-events-chemical-treatment/
article/466610/.

D'Amico, Anthony V. "Treatment and Monitoring for Early Prostate Cancer."
New England Journal of Medicine, October 13, 2016. http://www.nejm.org/
doi/full/10.1056/NEJMe1610395#t=article.

Dana-Farber Cancer Institute. "Sexual Health, Intimacy, and Cancer." Accessed
July 13, 2020. https://www.dana-farber.org.

Dana-Farber Cancer Institute. "Study Finds Upsurge in 'Active Surveillance'
for Low-risk Prostate Cancer." News release, February 11, 2019. https://
www.dana-farber.org/newsroom/news-releases/2019/study-finds-upsurge
-in--active-surveillance--for-low-risk-prostate-cancer/.

DiNicolantonio, James J., J. McCarty, Mark F; Levie, Carl, and James H.
O'Keefe. *Missouri Medicine*, July-August 2003. https://www.ncbi.nlm.nih
.gov/pmc/articles/PMC6179880/.

E

Emmons, Steve. "State of the Prostate." *Los Angeles Times*, March 7, 1997.
https://www.latimes.com/archives/la-xpm-1997-03-07-ls-35560-story.html.

Epstein, Nancy. "Multidisciplinary In-hospital Teams Improve Patient Outcomes: A Review." *Surgical Neurology International*, August 28, 2014.
https://www.ncbi.nlm.nih.gov/pmc/articles/PMC4173201/.

Etzioni, Ruth, Roman Gulati, Matt R. Cooperberg, David M. Penson et al.
"Limitations of Basing Screening Policies on Screening Trials: The US Pre-
ventive Services Task Force and Prostate Cancer Screening." *Medical Care*,
April 2013. https://pubmed.ncbi.nlm.nih.gov/23269114/.

Everyday Health. "9 Popular Ways to Treat Erectile Dysfunction." August 2019.
https://www.everydayhealth.com/erectile-dysfunction-pictures/popular
-ways-to-treat-erectile-dysfunction.aspx.

F

Fine, Rhonda. "Sexual Problems After Prostate Cancer." His Prostate Cancer.
July 31, 2019. https://www.hisprostatecancer.com/sexual-problems.html.

Fizazi, Karim, Michael Carducci, Matthew Smith, Ronaldo Damião et al.
"Denosumab versus Zoledronic Acid for Treatment of Bone Metastases
in Men with Castration-resistant Prostate Cancer: A Randomized, Double-
blind Study." *The Lancet*, February 25, 2011. https://pubmed.ncbi.nlm.nih
.gov/21353695/.

Free Dictionary. "Work-up." Accessed July 2010. https://www.thefreediction
ary.com/workup.

Future Medicine. "Prostate Cancer: Quality of Life, Psychosocial Implications and Treatment Choices." August 4, 2008. https://www.ncbi.nlm.nih.gov/pmc/articles/PMC2796196/.

G

Genetics Home Reference. "BRCA2 Gene." August 17, 2020. https://ghr.nlm.nih.gov/gene/BRCA2.

George, Nancie. "6 Superfoods for a Healthy Prostate." *Men's Health*, February 19, 2015. https://www.everydayhealth.com/pictures/superfoods-for-a-healthy-prostate/.

Gilbert, Bruce R. Northwell Health. May 2019. https://www.northwell.edu/find-care/find-a-doctor/urology/dr-bruce-r-gilbert-md-11308199.

Godwin, Jennifer. "Couples Counseling Boosts Sex Lives After Prostate Cancer." *HealthDay*, September 26, 2011. https://consumer.healthday.com/cancer-information-5/mis-cancer-news-102/couples-counseling-boosts-sex-lives-after-prostate-cancer-657217.html.

H

Harvard Health Letter. "Big Jump in Active Surveillance for Low-risk Prostate cancer." June 2019. https://www.health.harvard.edu/newsletter_article/big-jump-in-active-surveillance-for-low-risk-prostate-cancer.

Harvard Health Publishing. "A Patient's Story: Overcoming Incontinence." March 11, 2009. https://www.health.harvard.edu/blog/a-patients-story-overcoming-incontinence-2009031125.

Harvard Health Publishing. "New Options for Treating Erectile Dysfunction." March 11, 2009. https://www.harvardprostateknowledge.org/new-options-for-treating-erectile-dysfunction.

Harvard Health Publishing. "Study Investigates Treatment Regret Among Prostate Cancer Survivors." October 20, 2017. https://www.health.harvard.edu/blog/treatment-regret-prostate-cancer-2017102012535.

Harvard Health Publishing. "2020 Annual Report on Prostate Diseases," 52. https://www.health.harvard.edu/mens-health/2019-annual-report-on-prostate-diseases.

Harvard Health Publishing. "Types of Urinary Incontinence." December 2014. https://www.health.harvard.edu/bladder-and-bowel/types-of-urinary-incontinence.

Harvard University. "Does Prostate Cancer Screening Matter?" Annual Report. August 2017. https://www.health.harvard.edu/mens-health/does-prostate-cancer-screening-matter.

Harvard University. "Harvard Perspectives on Prostate Disease Prostate Cancer and Relationships: The Partner's Story." August 1, 2009. https://www.health

.harvard.edu/newsletter_article/Prostate-cancer-and-relationships-The
-partners-story.

Health Affairs. "Toward the 'Tipping Point': Decision Aids and Informed."
May/June 2007. https://www.healthaffairs.org/author/O%27Connor%2C+
Annette+M.

Healthline. "Anatomy and Function of Seminal Vesicles." July 30, 2018.
https://www.healthline.com/human-body-maps/seminal-vesicles/male.

Healthline. "Bone Metastasis: What Are the Symptoms?" April 1, 2019. https://
www.healthline.com/health/prostate-cancer-prognosis-life-expectancy-bone
-metastases#symptoms.

Healthline. "Sulforaphane: Side Effects and Food Sources, Benefits." February 26, 2019. https://www.healthline.com/nutrition/sulforaphane.

Healthline. "What Are Early Symptoms of Prostate Cancer?" March 28,
2017. https://www.healthline.com/health/prostate-cancer-symptoms#urinary
-symptoms.

Healthline. "What Happens When Prostate Cancer Spread to the Bones?"
Accessed July 15, 2020. https://www.healthline.com/health/prostate-cancer
-prognosis-life-expectancy-bone-metastases.

Heijnsdijk, E. A. M, A. der Kinderen, E. M. Wever et al. "Overdetection,
Overtreatment and Costs in Prostate-specific Antigen Screening for Prostate
Cancer." *British Journal of Cancer*, November 10, 2009. https://www.ncbi
.nlm.nih.gov/pmc/articles/PMC2788248.

Henry J. Kaiser Family Foundation "Population Distribution by Sex." Accessed
September 23, 2020. https://www.kff.org/.

Hoffman, Richard M. "Screening for Prostate Cancer." *UpToDate*, updated
March 2, 2020. Accessed August 12, 2020. https://www.uptodate.com/
contents/screening-for-prostate-cancer/print.

Hoffman, Richard M., Mary Lo, Jack A. Clark, Peter C. Albertsen et al. "Treatment Decision Regret Among Long-Term Survivors of Localized Prostate
Cancer: Results from the Prostate Cancer Outcomes Study." *Journal of
Clinical Oncology*, July 10, 2017. http://ascopubs.org/doi/abs/10.1200/JCO.
2016.70.6317?journalCode=jco.

Hu, Jim C., Paul Nguyen, and Jialin Mao. "Increase in Prostate Cancer Distant Metastases at Diagnosis in the United State." *Journal of the American Medical Association*, May 2017. xhttps://jamanetwork.com/journals/
jamaoncology/article-abstract/2594540.

Hugosson, Jonas, Sigrid Carlsson; Gunnar Aus; Svante Bergdahl et al. "Mortality Results from the Goteborg Randomised Population-based Prostate-Cancer Screening Trial." *The Lancet Oncology*, July 1, 2010. https://www
.thelancet.com/journals/lanonc/article/PIIS1470-2045(10)70146-7/fulltext.

Hugosson, Jonas, Sigrid V. Carlsson, Gunnar Aus, Svante Bergdahl et al. "PSA
Testing for Prostate Cancer Improves Survival—But Can We Do Better?"

The Lancet Oncology, August 11, 2010. https://www.thelancet.com/journals/lanonc/article/PIIS1470-2045%2810%2970152-2/fulltext.

Hugosson, Jonas, Rebecka Arnsrud Godtman, Sigrid V. Carlsson, Gunnar Aus et al. "Eighteen-year Follow-up of the Göteborg Randomized Population-based Prostate Cancer Screening Trial: Effect of Sociodemographic Variables on Participation, Prostate Cancer Incidence and Mortality." *Scandinavian Journal of Urology*, December 18, 2017. https://www.tandfonline.com/doi/abs/10.1080/21681805.2017.1411392.

Humanitas. "Why?" May 2019. https://www.humanitas.net/why-humanitas/.

I

InformedHealth.org. "How Does the Prostate Work?" August 23, 2016. https://www.ncbi.nlm.nih.gov/books/NBK279291/.

International Patient Decision Aid Standards Collaboration. May 31, 2019. http://ipdas.ohri.ca.

J

James, Susan Donaldson. "Prostate Cancer Counseling Helps Couples' Sex Lives, Says Study." ABC News, September 26, 2011. http://abcnews.go.com/Health/prostate-cancer-study-finds-couples-counseling-helps-restore/story?id=14592459.

Jennings, Dana. "Living with Incontinence After Prostate Cancer." *New York Times*, March 3, 2009. https://well.blogs.nytimes.com/2009/03/03/living-with-incontinence-after-prostate-cancer/.

Johns Hopkins Medicine. "Prostate Cancer and Diet." Winter 2000. http://urology.jhu.edu/newsletter/prostate_cancer512.php.

Johns Hopkins Medicine. "Erectile Dysfunction After Prostate Cancer." Accessed September 19, 2020. https://www.hopkinsmedicine.org/health/conditions-and-diseases/prostate-cancer/erectile-dysfunction-after-prostate-cancer.

Jones, Abigail. "Sex and Cancer: Why Is Nobody Talking About It?" *Newsweek*, July 17, 2017. http://www.newsweek.com/2017/07/28/cancer-sex-life-saving-treatments-havoc-intimacy-638396.html.

Jones, Miranda R., Corinne E. Joshu, Norma Kanarek, Ana Navas-Acien et al. "Cigarette Smoking and Prostate Cancer Mortality in Four States 1999–2010." *Preventing Chronic Disease*, April 14, 2016. https://www.cdc.gov/pcd/issues/2016/15_0454.htm.

K

Kantoff, Philip W., Celestia S. Higano, Neal D. Shore, E. Roy Berger et. al. "Sipuleucel-T Immunotherapy for Castration-Resistant Prostate Cancer."

New England Journal of Medicine, July 29, 2010. https://www.nejm.org/doi/full/10.1056/NEJMoa1001294.

KevinMD.com. "After Prostate Cancer Treatment: What about Intimacy for Men?" December 16, 2014. https://www.kevinmd.com/blog/2014/12/prostate-cancer-treatment-intimacy-men.html.

KevinMD.com. "How Politics Weakened the USPSTF." Accessed August 23, 2011. https://www.kevinmd.com/blog/2011/08/politics-weakened-uspstf.html.

Klein, Eric A. *Management of Prostate Cancer (Current Clinical Urology).* 2nd edition. New York: Humana Press, 2004, 481–89.

L

Live Science. "What Does the Prostate Do?" August 9, 2010. https://www.livescience.com/32751-what-does-the-prostate-gland-do.html.

M

Maeda, Yasuko, Morten Høyer, Lilli Lundby, and Christine Norton. "Faecal Incontinence Following Radiotherapy for Prostate Cancer: A Systematic Review." *Radiotherapy & Oncology*, January 24, 2011. https://www.thegreenjournal.com/article/S0167-8140(10)00724-3/fulltext.

Makarov, Danil V., Kristin Chrouser, John L. Gore, Jodi Maranchie et al. "AUA White Paper on Implementation of Shared Decision Making into Urological Practice." Science Direct, September 5, 2016. http://www.sciencedirect.com/science/article/pii/S2352077915002733.

Mandal, Dr. Amaya. "Semen Physiology." News: Medical Life Science. Updated February 27, 2019. https://www.news-medical.net/health/Semen-Physiology.aspx.

Mayo Clinic. "Intensity-modulated Radiation Therapy (IMRT)." Accessed September 10, 2020. https://www.mayoclinic.org/tests-procedures/intensity-modulated-radiation-therapy/about/pac-20385147.

Mayo Clinic. "Pomegranate Juice: A Cure for Prostate Cancer?" Accessed July 15, 2020. https://www.mayoclinic.org/diseases-conditions/prostate-cancer/expert-answers/pomegranate-juice/faq-20058204.

Mayo Clinic. "Prostate Biopsy." Accessed September 23, 2020. https://www.mayoclinic.org/tests-procedures/prostate-biopsy/about/pac-20384734.

Mayo Clinic. "Prostate Cancer, Diagnosis, Coping and Support," May 2019. https://www.mayoclinic.org/diseases-conditions/prostate-cancer/diagnosis-treatment/drc-20353093.

Mayo Clinic. "Prostate Cancer Metastasis: Where Does Prostate Cancer Spread." February 2, 2019. https://www.mayoclinic.org/diseases-conditions/prostate-cancer/expert-answers/prostate-cancer-metastasis/faq-20058270.

Mayo Clinic. "Ways to Reduce Your Risk—Prostate Cancer Prevention." November 6, 2018. https://www.mayoclinic.org/diseases-conditions/prostate-cancer/in-depth/prostate-cancer-prevention/art-20045641.

McIntosh, Hugh. "Why Do African-American Men Suffer More Prostate Cancer?" *Journal of the National Cancer Institute*, February 5, 1997. https://academic.oup.com/jnci/article/89/3/188/2526672.

MedHelp. "Leaving My Husband 4 Years After Prostate Cancer." November 22, 2009. https://www.medhelp.org/posts/Relationships/leaving-my-husband-4yrs-after-prostate-cancer/show/1108395.

Medical News Today. "Study Identifies Five Different Types of Prostate Cancer." July 30, 2015. https://www.medicalnewstoday.com/articles/297516.

Medical News Today. *"What is the prostate gland?"* January 11, 2018. https://www.medicalnewstoday.com/articles/319859.php.

MedicineNet. "Bowel Incontinence (Fecal Incontinence)" Accessed May 2019. https://www.medicinenet.com/fecal_incontinence/article.htm.

MedicineNet. "How Is Urinary Incontinence in Men Treated?" May 15, 2019. https://www.medicinenet.com/urinary_incontinence/article.htm#how_is_urinary_incontinence_ui_in_men_treated.

MedicineNet. "Urinary Incontinence in Men." May 15, 2019. https://www.medicinenet.com/urinary_incontinence/article.htm.

MedNet News. "Taking the Bias Out of Prostate Cancer." March 12, 2020. https://www.mednetnews.com/2020/03/12/multid-taking-the-bias-out-of-prostate-cancer-tx/.

MedPage Today. "Message on Prostate Surgery Results Not Getting Through." August 10, 2011. https://www.medpagetoday.com/hematologyoncology/prostatecancer/27977.

MedScape, "In NYC Subway, CyberKnife Prostate Cancer Ads Mislead." Accessed May 6, 2019. https://www.medscape.com/viewarticle/912619.

Memorial Sloan Kettering Cancer Center. "Inherited Risk for Prostate Cancer." April 15, 2013. https://www.mskcc.org/cancer-care/risk-assessment-screening/hereditary-genetics/genetic-counseling/inherited-risk-prostate.

Men's Hormonal Health. "What Are Normal PSA Levels by Age." June 23, 2019. https://www.menshormonalhealth.com/psa-test-results.html.

Mitchell, Jacqueline. "Flip the Switch." Harvard Medical School. January 15, 2018. https://hms.harvard.edu/news/flip-switch#.WmAO302sF34.mailto.

Mushroom-Appreciation.com. "So, What Are Some Different Types of Mushrooms?" Accessed July 15, 2020. https://www.mushroom-appreciation.com/types-of-mushrooms.html#sthash.UQal4Vud.yJqV63I8.dpbs.

N

National Cancer Institute. "Metastatic Cancer." Accessed July 15, 2020. https://www.cancer.gov/types/metastatic-cancer.

National Cancer Institute. "NCI-Designated Cancer Centers." June 24, 2019. https://www.cancer.gov/research/nci-role/cancer-centers.

National Cancer Institute. "SEER Cancer Statistics Review 1975–2004." Accessed on October 16, 2009. https://seer.cancer.gov/archive/csr/1975_2004/.

Nelson, Roxanne. "Preserving Intimacy After Prostate Cancer." Fred Hutch, May 13, 2014. https://www.fredhutch.org/en/news/center-news/2014/05/Intimacy-after-prostate-cancer.html.

O

Oncology Learning Network. "Current Guidelines Unreliable for Detecting Germline Variants in Prostate Cancer." March 2019. https://www.oncnet.com/news/current-guidelines-unreliable-detecting-germline-variants-prostate-cancer.

OncLive. "Task Force Changes Stance on Value of PSA Test." May 2018. https://www.onclive.com/publications/oncology-live/2018/vol-19-no-11/task-force-changes-stance-on-value-of-psa-test.

P

Pagan, Camille Noe. "Advanced Prostate Cancer and Your Relationship." *Web*MD, December 10, 2016. https://www.webmd.com/prostate-cancer/advanced-prostate-cancer-16/relationship-intimacy.

Pagan, Camille Noe. "Palliative Care for Advanced Prostate Cancer." *Web*MD, December 10, 2016. https://www.webmd.com/prostate-cancer/advanced-prostate-cancer-16/prostate-cancer-palliative-care.

Paul, Marla. "Metastatic Prostate Cancer Cases Way Up, Increase May Be Due to More Lax Screening or More Aggressive Disease." Northwestern Now. July 19, 2016. https://news.northwestern.edu/stories/2016/07/metastatic-prostate-cancer-cases-skyrocket.

Persaud, Natasha. "Prostate Cancer Screening Recommendations." *Updates Renal & Urology News*, May 8, 2018. https://www.renalandurologynews.com/prostate-cancer/uspstf-updates-prostate-cancer-screening-recommendations/article/764254/.

Prostate Cancer Foundation. "Immunotherapy: A Vaccine for Prostate Cancer." June 15, 2017. https://www.pcf.org/news/immunotherapy-a-vaccine-for-prostate-cancer/.

Prostate Cancer Foundation. "Prostate Cancer Additional Facts for African American Men and Their Families." Accessed July 15, 2020. https://res.cloudinary.com/pcf/image/upload/v1553031384/AfAm_PCaInfoGuide-031919_dygfjz.pdf.

Prostate Cancer Foundation. "Prostate Cancer Guide." Accessed July 15, 2020. https://www.pcf.org/guide/.

Prostate Cancer Foundation. "The Science of Living Well, Beyond Cancer." 2019. https://res.cloudinary.com/pcf/image/upload/v1574120581/Wellness Guide_interactive_rev11.15.19_goostr.pdf.

ProstateCancer.net. "Types of Prostate Cancer." November 11, 2017. https://prostatecancer.net/basics/types/.

Prostate.net. "What Are Late Stage Prostate Cancer Symptoms." January 17, 2019, https://prostate.net/what-are-late-stage-prostate-cancer-symptoms/.

Prostate Cancer UK, "Your Diet and Physical Activity." July 15, 2020. https://prostatecanceruk.org/prostate-information/living-with-prostate-cancer/your-diet-and-physical-activity.

Q

Quinn, M., and P. Babb. "Patterns and Trends in Prostate Cancer Incidence, Survival, Prevalence and Mortality. Part 1: International Comparisons." *BJUI International*, June 24, 2002. https://onlinelibrary.wiley.com/doi/full/10.1046/j.1464-410X.2002.2822.x.

R

Rapaport, Lisa. "Blacks with Prostate Cancer Less Likely to Get Ideal Treatment." August 23, 2017. https://www.reuters.com/article/us-prostate-treatment-race/blacks-with-prostate-cancer-less-likely-to-get-ideal-treatment-idUSKCN1B32E6.

Redner, Rick. "8 Reasons Why Sexual Desire Is Reduced After Prostate Surgery." *Prostate Cancer News Today*, August 4, 2017. https://prostatecancernewstoday.com/2017/08/04/prostate-cancer-surgery-eight-reasons-why-sexual-desire-is-reduced/.

Renal & Urology News. "Prostate Cancer Screening Recommendations." May 8, 2018. https://www.renalandurologynews.com/prostate-cancer/uspstf-updates-prostate-cancer-screening-recommendations/article/764254/.

S

Sanda, Martin G., Rodney L. Dunn, Jeff Michalski, Howard M. Sandler et al. "Quality of Life and Satisfaction with Outcome Among Prostate-Cancer Survivors." *New England Journal of Medicine*, March 20, 2008. https://www.ncbi.nlm.nih.gov/pubmed/18354103.

Sanford, Melissa T., Kirsten L. Greene, and Peter R. Carroll. "The Argument for Palliative Care in Prostate Cancer." *Translational Andrology and Urology*, December 2, 2013. https://www.ncbi.nlm.nih.gov/pmc/articles/PMC4708113/.

Schmidt, Charles. "Using PSA to Determine Prognosis." Harvard Health Publishing, November 17, 2009. https://www.health.harvard.edu/blog/using-psa-to-determine-prognosis-20091117168.

Schröder, Fritz H., Jonas Hugosson, Sigrid Carlsson, Maciej Kwiatkowski et. al. "Screening for Prostate Cancer Decreases the Risk of Developing Metastatic Disease: Findings from the European Randomized Study of Screening for Prostate Cancer (ERSPC)." *European Urology*, June 11, 2012. https://www.europeanurology.com/article/S0302-2838(12)00687-2/fulltext/ screening-for-prostate-cancer-decreases-the-risk-of-developing-metastatic -disease-findings-from-the-european-randomized-study-of-screening-for -prostate-cancer-erspc.

Schröder, F. H., J. Hugosson, M. J. Roobol et al. "Prostate-cancer Mortality at 11 Years of Follow-up." *New England Journal of Medicine*, March 15, 2012. https://pubmed.ncbi.nlm.nih.gov/22417251/.

Schröder, F. H., J. Hugosson, M. J. Roobol et al. "Screening and prostate-cancer mortality in a randomized European study." *New England Journal of Medicine*, March 26, 2009. https://www.nejm.org/doi/full/10.1056/ NEJMoa0810084.

Science Daily. "Eating Mushrooms May Help Lower Prostate Cancer." September 5, 2009, https://www.sciencedaily.com/releases/2019/09/190905080106 .htm.

Science Daily. "Starving Prostate Cancer with What You Eat: Apple Peels, Red Grapes, Turmeric." June 6, 2017. https://www.sciencedaily.com/ releases/2017/06/170606112750.htm.

Siegel, Rebecca L., and Kimberly D. Miller. "Cancer Statistics, 2017." *CA: Cancer Journal for Clinicians*, January 5, 2017. https://onlinelibrary.wiley .com/doi/full/10.3322/caac.21387.

Smith, Matthew R., Fred Saad, Robert Coleman, Neal Shore et al. "Denosumab and Bone-Metastasis-Free Survival in Men with Castration-Resistant Prostate Cancer: Results of a Phase 3, Randomized, Placebo-Controlled Trial." *The Lancet*, November 16, 2011. https://www.thelancet.com/journals/lancet/ article/PIIS0140-6736(11)61226-9/fulltext.

Snedecor, Sonya J., John A Carter, Satyin Kaura, and Marc F Botteman. "Denosumab Versus Zoledronic Acid for Treatment of Bone Metastases in Men with Castration-Resistant Prostate Cancer: A Randomized, Double-blind Study." *Journal of Medical Economics*, September 5, 2012. https:// pubmed.ncbi.nlm.nih.gov/22870908/.

Sonoda, Tomoko, Yoshie Nagata, Mitsuru Mori, Naoto Miyanaga et al. "A Case-control Study of Diet and Prostate Cancer in Japan; Possible Protective Effect of Traditional Japanese Diet." *Cancer Science*, August 19, 2005. https://onlinelibrary.wiley.com/doi/abs/10.1111/j.1349-7006.2004. tb02209.x.

STAT. "Long-term Study Shows Most Prostate Cancer Patients Don't Need Aggressive Treatment." December 12, 2018. https://www.statnews

.com/2018/12/12/long-term-study-prostate-cancer-patients-dont-need-treat
ment/.

Sweeny, Christopher, Yu-Hui Chen, Michael Anthony Carducci, Glenn Liu et
al. "Impact on Overall Survival with Chemohormonal Therapy Versus Hormonal Therapy for Home-Sensitivity Newly Metastatic Prostate Cancer: An
ECOG-led phase III randomized trial." *Journal of Clinical Oncology*, January 31, 2017. https://ascopubs.org/doi/abs/10.1200/jco.2014.32.18_suppl
.lba2.

T

Tannock, Ian F., Ronald de Wit, William R. Berry, Jozsef Horti et al.
"Docetaxel plus Prednisone or Mitoxantrone plus Prednisone for Advanced
Prostate Cancer." *New England Journal of Medicine*, October 7, 2004.
https://www.nejm.org/doi/full/10.1056/NEJMoa040720.

Tempany, Clare M. C., Peter R. Carroll, and Michael S. Leapman. "The Role of
Magnetic Resonance Imaging in Prostate Cancer." *UpToDate*, January 20,
2020. https://www.uptodate.com/contents/the-role-of-magnetic-resonance
-imaging-in-prostate-cancer.

Texas Oncology. "Recurrent Prostate Cancer." Accessed July 13, 2020. https://
www.texasoncology.com/types-of-cancer/prostate-cancer/recurrent-prostate
-cancer.

U

United Kingdom National Health Service. "PSA Testing." June 12, 2021.
https://www.nhs.uk/conditions/prostate-cancer/psa-testing/.

University of California-Los Angeles Health. "Dealing with Erectile Dysfunction." Accessed July 18, 2020. https://www.uclahealth.org/urology/
prostate-cancer/dealing-with-erectile-dysfunction.

University of California-San Francisco Health. "Patient's Guide to Prostate
Cancer: Treatments." July 2019. https://www.ucsfhealth.org/education/
patients_guide_to_prostate_cancer/treatments/.

University of California-San Francisco. "Prostate Cancer & Its Treatment: Section VI Treatment Options." Accessed September 10, 2020. https://campus
lifeservices.ucsf.edu/dmx/PatientEd/SDURO0080.pdf.

University of California-San Francisco. "Prostate Cancer Treatments, New
Treatments and Clinical Trials." April 2019. https://www.ucsfhealth.org/
conditions/prostate_cancer/treatment.html.

University of California-San Francisco Health. "Psycho-Oncology." Accessed
July 20, 2019. https://www.ucsfhealth.org/services/psycho-oncology/.

University of Massachusetts Medical School Department of Urology. "Salvage Prostatectomy." Accessed July 11, 2020. https://www.umassmed.edu/
urology/clinical-conditions/cancer/salvage-prostatectomy/.

University of Texas Southwestern Medical Center. "The Power of Cascade Testing." December 30, 2015. http://www.utswmedicine.org/stories/articles/year-2015/cascade-testing.html.

UpToDate. "Cancer Statistics 2017." January 2017. https://pubmed.ncbi.nlm .nih.gov/28055103/.

UpToDate. "Screening for Prostate Cancer." Updated March 2, 2020. https:// www.uptodate.com/contents/screening-for-prostate-cancer.

UpToDate. "The Role of Magnetic Resonance Imaging in Prostate Cancer." January 20, 2020. https://www.uptodate.com/contents/the-role-of-magnetic -resonance-imaging-in-prostate-cancer.

U.S. Preventive Services Task Force. "Prostate Cancer: Screening." May 8, 2018. https://www.uspreventiveservicestaskforce.org/Page/Document/ UpdateSummaryFinal/prostate-cancer-screening.

U.S. Preventive Services Task Force. "Prostate Cancer Treatments." Accessed July 13, 2020. https://www.ucsfhealth.org/conditions/prostate_cancer/treat ment.html.

U.S. Preventive Services Task Force. "Screening for Prostate Cancer." July 17, 2012. https://pubmed.ncbi.nlm.nih.gov/22801674/.

USTOO.com. "Learn to Fight Prostate Cancer." Accessed September 11, 2020. https://www.ustoo.org.

V

von Radowitz, John. "Tall Men Are More Likely to Develop Prostate Cancer, New Research Suggests." *The Independent,* July 13, 2017. https:// www.independent.co.uk/life-style/health-and-families/health-news/prostate -cancer-tall-men-increased-risk-disease-death-tumours-height-correlation -oxford-university-a7838481.html.

W

*Web*MD, "A Partner's Guide to Erectile Dysfunction," Marianne Wait, December 13, 2015, https://www.webmd.com/erectile-dysfunction/features/a -womans-guide-to-ed.

*Web*MD, "If Your Partner Has ED," Reviewed by Nazia Q. Bandukwala, DO, February 11, 2020, https://www.webmd.com/erectile-dysfunction/guide/ ed-supporting-your-partner.

*Web*MD. "Is There a Prostate Cancer Diet?" Accessed July 15, 2020. https:// www.webmd.com/prostate-cancer/features/is-there-prostate-cancer-diet.

*Web*MD. "Palliative Care for Advanced Prostate Cancer." Accessed July 13, 2020. https://www.webmd.com/prostate-cancer/prostate-cancer-palliative -care#1.

*Web*MD. "Prostate Cancer: Laparoscopic Prostate Surgery." December 2019. www.webmd.com/prostate-cancer/guide/laparoscopic-prostate-surgery#1.

*Web*MD. "Types of Prostate Disease." Accessed July 11, 2020. https://www.webmd.com/prostate-cancer/symptoms-types-prostate-cancer.

*Web*MD. "What Are Kegels, and Why Should I Do Them?" Accessed July 13, 2020. https://www.webmd.com/women/guide/kegels-should-i-do-them.

*Web*MD. "What Is Metastatic Prostate Cancer." April 22, 2019. https://www.webmd.com/prostate-cancer/metastatic-prostate-cancer#1.

*Web*MD. "What Is Metastatic Prostate Cancer?" Accessed July 15, 2020. https://www.webmd.com/prostate-cancer/advanced-prostate-cancer-16/metastatic-prostate-cancer.

Web Physicians. "Pre-op Counseling for Prostate Surgery Not Effective." January 3, 2012. http://urology.webphysicians.org/2012/01/03/pre-op-counseling-for-prostate-surgery-not-effective/.

Weill Cornell School of Medicine. "Incidence of Metastatic Prostate Cancer in Older Men Increases Following Drop in PSA Screening." December 29, 2016. https://news.weill.cornell.edu/news/2016/12/incidence-of-metastatic-prostate-cancer-in-older-men-increases-following-drop-in-psa.

Weiner, A. B., R. S. Matulewicz, S. E. Eggener, and E. M. Schaeffer. "Increasing Incidence of Prostate Cancer in the United States (2004–2013)." *Prostate Cancer and Prostatic Diseases*, July 19, 2016. https://www.nature.com/articles/pcan201630.

Weintraub, Karen. "Long-term Study Shows Most Prostate Cancer Patients Don't Need Aggressive Treatment." *STAT*, December 12, 2018.

Welch, H. G., and P. C. Albertsen. "U.S. Preventive Services Task Force Recommendation Statement." *Journal of the National Cancer Institute*, October 7, 2009. https://pubmed.ncbi.nlm.nih.gov/19720969/.

World Cancer Research Fund International. "Our Analysis of Worldwide Research on Prostate Cancer." November 19, 2014. "http://www.wcrf.org/int/research-we-fund/continuous-update-project-findings-reports/prostate-cancer.

World Health Organization. "Definition of Palliative Care." Accessed July 13, 2020. http://www.who.int/cancer/palliative/definition/en/.

Z

Zauber, Ann G., Iris Lansdorp-Vogelaar, Amy B. Knudsen, and Janneke Wilschut. "Evaluating Test Strategies for Colorectal Cancer Screening: A Decision Analysis for the U.S. Preventive Services Task Force." *Annals of Internal Medicine*, November 4, 2008.

Zelman, Kathleen. "Diet and Weight Loss." October 27, 2016. https://www.medicinenet.com/diet_weight_loss_sugar/article.htm?ecd=mnl_spc_071819.

ZERO Cancer. "Fatigue." Accessed May 2019. https://zerocancer.org/learn/current-patients/side-effects/fatigue/.

ZERO Cancer. "Life After Treatment." Accessed July 13, 2020. https://zero cancer.org/learn/survivors/life-after-treatment/.

ZERO Cancer. "Recurrence." Accessed July 13, 2020. https://zerocancer.org/ learn/survivors/recurrence/.

Zhang, Kai, Chris H. Bankgma, and Monique J. Roobol. "Prostate Cancer Screening in Europe and Asia." *Asian Journal of Urology*, April 2017. http:// www.sciencedirect.com/science/article/pii/S2214388216300558.

Notes

Introduction

1. "Key Statistics for Prostate Cancer," American Cancer Society, accessed November 11, 2020, https://www.cancer.org/cancer/prostate-cancer/about/key-statistics.html.
2. "Find a Doctor," Dana-Farber Cancer Institute, accessed November 11, 2020, https://www.dana-farber.org/find-a-doctor/sharon-bober/.
3. Michael O. Schroeder, "How Can Men Lower Their Risk of Dying from Prostate Cancer?" U.S. News, June 21, 2018, accessed November 11, 2020, https://health.usnews.com/health-care/patient-advice/articles/2018-06-21/how-can-men-lower-their-risk-of-dying-from-prostate-cancer.

Chapter 1

1. "Who Is at Risk for Prostate Cancer?" Centers for Disease Control and Prevention, accessed August 10, 2020, https://www.cdc.gov/cancer/prostate/basic_info/risk_factors.htm.

Chapter 2

1. "YouTube Has 1.8 Billion Logged-in Viewers Each Month," The Verge, May 3, 2018, accessed November 11, 2020, https://www.theverge.com/2018/5/3/17317274/youtube-1-8-billion-logged-in-monthly-users-brandcast-2018.
2. Charles Bankhead, "YouTube Videos Often Mislead on Prostate Cancer," MedPageToday, November 28, 2018, accessed November 12, 2020, https://www.medpagetoday.com/hematologyoncology/prostatecancer/76566.

3. "Dissemination of Misinformative and Biased Information about Prostate Cancer on YouTube," *European Urology*, November 27, 2018, accessed November 12, 2020, https://www.europeanurology.com/article/S0302-2838(18)30854-6/fulltext.

Chapter 3

1. "Key Statistics for Prostate Cancer," About Prostate Cancer, American Cancer Society, accessed on November 12, 2020, https://www.cancer.org/cancer/prostate-cancer/about/key-statistics.html.
2. "Prostate Cancer: A Guide for Aging Men," Aging.com, accessed November 13, 2020, https://aging.com/prostate-cancer-a-guide-for-aging-men/.
3. Dr. Richard M. Hoffman, "Screening for Prostate Cancer," UpToDate, accessed November 12, 2020, https://www.uptodate.com/contents/screening-for-prostate-cancer/print.

Chapter 4

1. "Types of Prostate Cancer," November 11, 2017, https://prostatecancer.net/basics/types/.
2. "Study identifies five different types of prostate cancer," *Medical News Today*, July 30, 2015, https://www.medicalnewstoday.com/articles/297516.
3. "Signs and Symptoms of Prostate Cancer," American Cancer Society, August 1, 2019, https://www.cancer.org/cancer/prostate-cancer/detection-diagnosis-staging/signs-symptoms.html.
4. "Types of Prostate Cancer," *Web*MD, accessed July 11, 2010, https://www.webmd.com/prostate-cancer/symptoms-types-prostate-cancer.
5. Ibid.
6. "Prostate Cancer Symptoms," American Cancer Society, accessed July 11, 2020, https://www.webmd.com/prostate-cancer/guide/understanding-prostate-cancer-symptoms.

Chapter 5

1. Kenneth Lin, "How politics weakened the USPSTF," KevinMD.com, August 23, 2011, https://www.kevinmd.com/blog/2011/08/politics-weakened-uspstf.html.
2. Ibid.
3. "Early Detection of Prostate Cancer: AUA Guideline," *Journal of Urology*, August 1, 2013, 19, https://www.auajournals.org/doi/full/10.1016/j.juro.2013.04.119.

4. Ibid., 14, 15.

5. Ibid., 16.

6. "Taking the Bias Out of Prostate Cancer," MedNet News, March 12, 2020, https://www.mednetnews.com/2020/03/12/multid-taking-the-bias-out-of -prostate-cancer-tx/.

7. Karen Weintraub, "Long-term Study Shows Most Prostate Cancer Patients Don't Need Aggressive Treatment," Stat newsletter, December 12, 2018, https://www.statnews.com/2018/12/12/long-term-study-prostate-cancer -patients-dont-need-treatment/.

8. "Early Detection of Prostate Cancer 2018," American Urological Association, 2013, https://www.auanet.org/guidelines/prostate-cancer-early -detection-guideline.

9. "Does Prostate Cancer Screening Matter?" "Harvard Men's Health Watch," Harvard University, August 2017, https://www.health.harvard.edu/ mens-health/does-prostate-cancer-screening-matter.

10. Ibid.

11. Dana-Farber Cancer Institute is a comprehensive cancer treatment and research center located in Boston. It is a teaching affiliate of Harvard Medical School and a founding member of the Dana-Farber/Harvard Cancer Center, designated as a Comprehensive Cancer Center by the National Cancer Institute.

12. "Screening for Prostate Cancer," *UpToDate*, last updated March 2, 2020, https://www.uptodate.com/contents/screening-for-prostate-cancer.

13. L. A. F. Ries, D. Melbert, M. Krapcho, A. Mariotto et al., SEER Cancer Statistics Review: 1975-2004, National Cancer Institute, accessed on October 16, 2009, http://seer.cancer.gov/csr/1975_2004/.

14. "Study Finds Upsurge in 'Active Surveillance' for Low-Risk Prostate Cancer," Dana-Farber news release, February 11, 2019, https://www .dana-farber.org/newsroom/news-releases/2019/study-finds-upsurge-in--active -surveillance--for-low-risk-prostate-cancer/.

Chapter 6

1. Anthony V. D'Amico, "Treatment and Monitoring for Early Prostate Cancer," *New England Journal of Medicine*, October 13, 2016, http://www .nejm.org/doi/full/10.1056/NEJMe1610395#t=article.

2. Ibid.

3. "Prostate Cancer Metastasis: Where Does Prostate Cancer Spread," Mayo Clinic, February 02, 2019, https://www.mayoclinic.org/diseases-conditions/ prostate-cancer/expert-answers/prostate-cancer-metastasis/faq-20058270.

4. "What Is Metastatic Cancer," *Web*MD, April 22, 2019.

5. "Bone Metastasis, What Are the Symptoms," Healthline.com, April 1, 2019, https://www.healthline.com/health/prostate-cancer-prognosis-life -expectancy-bone-metastases#symptoms.

6. "2016, Life Expectancy at Birth, at Age 65. . .," Health, United States, 2016, Table 15, Centers for Disease Control, May 2017, accessed November 13, 2020, https://www.cdc.gov/nchs/data/hus/hus16.pdf#015.

7. "Prostate Cancer: Screening," US Preventive Services Task Force, May 8, 2018, accessed November 13, 2020, https://www.uspreventiveservicestask force.org/Page/Document/UpdateSummaryFinal/prostate-cancer-screening.

8. Ibid., 3.

9. "Insurance Coverage for Prostate Cancer Screening," American Cancer Society, August 1, 2019.

10. Ibid.

11. "Big Jump in Active Surveillance for Low-Risk Prostate Cancer," Harvard Health Letter, June 2019, https://www.health.harvard.edu/newsletter_article/ big-jump-in-active-surveillance-for-low-risk-prostate-cancer.

12. Ibid.

Chapter 7

1. Charles Bankhead, "15 Percent of Men Regret Prostate Cancer Treatment Choices Years Later, Study Finds," STAT, July 12, 2017, https://www .statnews.com/2017/07/12/prostate-cancer-treatment-regret/.

2. Richard M. Hoffman, Mary Lo, Jack A. Clark, Peter C. Albertsen et al., "Treatment Decision Regret Among Long-Term Survivors of Localized Prostate Cancer: Results from the Prostate Cancer Outcomes Study," *Journal of Clinical Oncology*, July 2017, http://ascopubs.org/doi/abs/10.1200/JCO.2016 .70.6317?journalCode=jco.

3. "Mark P.," Patient Stories, Cancer Treatment Centers of America, accessed July 13, 2020, https://www.cancercenter.com/patient-stories/markp.

4. Ibid.

5. "The role of magnetic resonance imaging in prostate cancer," UpToDate, January 20, 2020, https://www.uptodate.com/contents/the-role-of-magnetic-res onance-imaging-in-prostate-cancer.

6. "Salvage Prostatectomy," Department of Urology, University of Massachusetts Medical School, accessed July 11, 2020, https://www.umassmed.edu/ urology/clinical-conditions/cancer/salvage-prostatectomy/.

7. H. Gilbert Welch and Peter C. Albertsen, "Prostate Cancer Diagnosis and Treatment After the Introduction of Prostate-Specific Antigen Screen: 1986–2005," *Journal of the National Cancer Institute*, October 7, 2009, https:// pubmed.ncbi.nlm.nih.gov/19720969/.

8. Virginia A. Moyer, "Screening for Prostate Cancer: U.S. Preventive Services Task Force Recommendation Statement," July 17, 2012, https://pubmed .ncbi.nlm.nih.gov/22801674/.

9. Martin G. Sanda, Rodney L. Dunn, Jeff Michalski, Howard M. Sandler et al., "Quality of Life and Satisfaction with Outcome Among Prostate-Cancer Survivors," *New England Journal of Medicine*, March 20, 2008, https://www .ncbi.nlm.nih.gov/pubmed/18354103.

Chapter 8

1. "Early Detection of Prostate Cancer, 2018," American Urological Association, Reviewed and Validity Confirmed 2018, http://www.auanet.org/ guidelines/prostate-cancer-early-detection-guideline.

2. Ibid.

3. E. A. M. Heijnsdijk, A. der Kinderen, E. M. Wever et al., "Overdetection, Overtreatment and Costs in Prostate-specific Antigen Screening for Prostate Cancer," *British Journal of Cancer*, November 10, 2009.

4. Ruth Etzioni, Roman Gulati, Matt R. Cooperberg et al.,"Limitations of basing screening policies on screening trials: The US Preventive Services Task Force and prostate cancer screening," National Center for Biotechnology Information, April 2013, https://pubmed.ncbi.nlm.nih.gov/23269114/.

5. "Prostate Cancer: Age-Specific Screening Guidelines," Health Conditions and Diseases, accessed November 13, 2020. https://www.hopkinsmedi cine.org/health/conditions-and-diseases/prostate-cancer/prostate-cancer-age -specific-screening-guidelines

6. "Test ID: PSA Diagnostic, Serum," Mayo Clinic Laboratories, accessed November 13, 2020, https://www.mayocliniclabs.com/test-catalog/ Clinical+and+Interpretive/9284.

7. "What Are Normal PSA Levels by Age," June 23, 2019, *Men's Hormonal Health*, https://www.menshormonalhealth.com/psa-test-results.html.

8. "Tests to Diagnose and Stage Prostate Cancer," American Cancer Society, accessed November 13, 2020, https://www.cancer.org/cancer/prostate -cancer/detection-diagnosis-staging/how-diagnosed.html.

9. "Prostate Biopsy," Patient Care and Health Information, Mayo Clinic, accessed November 13, 2020, https://www.mayoclinic.org/tests-procedures/ prostate-biopsy/about/pac-20384734.

10. "What are Seminal Vesicles and What Is Their Purpose?" Healthline, accessed November 13, 2020, https://www.healthline.com/human-body-maps/ seminal-vesicles/male.

11. "Tests to Diagnose and Stage Prostate Cancer, American Cancer Society, accessed November 13, 2020, https://www.cancer.org/cancer/prostate-cancer/detection-diagnosis-staging/how-diagnosed.html.

12. "Lymph Nodes," Cancer Treatment Centers of America, November 13, 2020, https://www.cancercenter.com/terms/lymph-nodes/.

13. "2020 Annual Report on Prostate Cancer," Harvard Health Publishing, November 13, 2020, 52, https://www.health.harvard.edu/mens-health/2019-annual-report-on-prostate-diseases.

14. "Using PSA to Determine Prognosis," Harvard Health Publishing, November 17, 2009, https://www.health.harvard.edu/blog/using-psa-to-determine-prognosis-20091117168.

15. "Prostate Cancer Patient Guide," Prostate Cancer Foundation, 65, https://www.pcf.org.

16. "The Power of Cascade Testing," UT Southwestern, December 30, 2015, accessed July 2020, http://www.utswmedicine.org/stories/articles/year-2015/cascade-testing.html.

17. "Current Guidelines Unreliable for Detecting GermlineVariants in Prostate Cancer," Oncology Learning Network, March 2019, https://www.oncnet.com/news/current-guidelines-unreliable-detecting-germline-variants-prostate-cancer.

Chapter 9

1. "Key Statistics for Prostate Cancer," American Cancer Society, 2019, accessed November 13, 2020, https://www.cancer.org/cancer/prostate-cancer/about/key-statistics.html.

2. Ibid.

3. "Early Detection of Prostate Cancer: AUA Guideline," American Urological Association, April 13, accessed November 13, 2020, https://phpa.health.maryland.gov/cancer/SiteAssets/SitePages/homemos/ccpc13-22--att4_AUA-Prostate-Cancer-Detection.pdf.

4. 2017 Annual Report on Prostate Cancer, Harvard University, 8.

5. "First Recommendation Statement: Prostate Cancer: Screening," United States Preventive Services Task Force, May 8, 2018, accessed November 13, 2020, https://www.uspreventiveservicestaskforce.org/Page/Document/UpdateSummaryFinal/prostate-cancer-screening.

6. Jason Harris, "Task Force Changes Stance on Value of PSA Test," Oncology Live, May 21, 2018, https://www.onclive.com/publications/oncology-live/2018/vol-19-no-11/task-force-changes-stance-on-value-of-psa-test.

7. "USPSTF Updates Prostate Cancer Screening Recommendations," Renal & Urology News, May 8, 2018, https://www.renalandurologynews.com/

prostate-cancer/uspstf-updates-prostate-cancer-screening-recommendations/article/764254/.

8. Maggie Fox, "Cases of Aggressive Prostate Cancer on the Rise," NBC News, July 19, 2016, accessed November 20, 2012, https://www.nbcnews.com/health/mens-health/cases-aggressive-prostate-cancer-rise-research-finds-n612661.

9. Fritz H. Schröder, Jonas Hugosson, Sigrid Carlsson et al., "Screening for Prostate Cancer Decreases the Risk of Developing Metastatic Disease: Findings from the European Randomized Study of Screening for Prostate Cancer (ERSPC)," *European Urology*, June 11, 2012, https://www.europeanurology.com/article/S0302-2838(12)00687-2/fulltext/screening-for-prostate-cancer-decreases-the-risk-of-developing-metastatic-disease-findings-from-the-european-randomized-study-of-screening-for-prostate-cancer-erspc.

10. F. H. Schroder, J. Hugosson, M. J. Roobol et al., "Screening and prostate-cancer mortality in a randomized European study," *New England Journal of Medicine*, March 26, 2009, https://www.nejm.org/doi/full/10.1056/NEJMoa0810084.

11. J. Hugosson, S. Carlsson, G. Aus et al., "Mortality Results from the Goteborg Randomised Population-based Prostate-Cancer Screening Trial," *Lancet Oncology* 11 (2010): 725–32, https://www.thelancet.com/journals/lanonc/article/PIIS1470-2045(10)70146-7/references.

12. Schroder, Hugosson, Roobol et al., "Screening and Prostate-Cancer Mortality in a Randomized European Study."

13. "Early Detection of Prostate Cancer, 2018," *American Urology Journal*, https://www.auanet.org/guidelines/prostate-cancer-early-detection-guideline.

14. "Survival Rates for Prostate Cancer," American Cancer Society, accessed July 2020, https://www.cancer.org/cancer/prostate-cancer/detection-diagnosis-staging/survival-rates.html.

15. Schröder, Hugosson, Carlsson et al., "Screening for Prostate Cancer Decreases the Risk of Developing Metastatic Disease."

16. Ibid.

17. A. G. Zauber, I. Lansdorp-Vogelaar, A. B. Knudsen et al., "Evaluating Test Strategies for Colorectal Cancer Screening: a Decision Analysis for the U.S. Preventive Services Task Force," *Annals of Internal Medicine*, October 6, 2008.

18. "Prostate Cancer Screening in Europe and Asia," *Asian Journal of Urology* 4, no. 2 (April 2017): 86–95, http://www.sciencedirect.com/science/article/pii/S2214388216300558.

19. "Early Detection of Prostate Cancer, Prostate-Cancer-Detection," American Urological Association, 2015, 12.

20. "Eighteen-Year Follow-Up of the Goteborg Randomized Population-Based Prostate Cancer Screening Trial," *Scandinavian Journal of Urology*,

vol. 52, no. 1 (2018), https://www.tandfonline.com/doi/abs/10.1080/21681805
.2017.1411392.

21. "Prostate Cancer Screening in Europe and Asia," *Asian Journal of Urology.*

22. "Prostate Cancer Screening," *British Journal of Urological Surgeons*, March 10, 2015, https://www.baus.org.uk/professionals/baus_business/publications/21/prostate_cancer_screening.

23. Hugosson, Carlsson, Aus et al., "Mortality Results from the Göteborg Randomised Population-based Prostate-Cancer Screening Trial"; D. E. Neal, "PSA Testing for Prostate Cancer Improves Survival—But Can We Do Better?" *Lancet Oncology* 11 (2010): 702–3, https://www.thelancet.com/journals/lanonc/article/PIIS1470-2045(10)70152-2/fulltext.

24. "Screening for Prostate Cancer," *UpToDate*, September 24, 2017, https://www.uptodate.com/contents/screening-for-prostate-cancer.

25. Schroder, Hugosson, Carlsson et al., "Screening for Prostate Cancer Decreases the Risk of Developing Metastatic Disease."

26. Schroder, Hugosson, Roobol et al., "Screening and Prostate-Cancer Mortality in a Randomized European Study."

27. Fritz H. Schroder, Jonas Hugosson, Monique. J. Roobol, Teuvo L. Tammela et al., "Prostate-cancer Mortality at 11 Years of Follow-up," *New England Journal of Medicine*, May 31, 2012, https://pubmed.ncbi.nlm.nih.gov/22417251/.

28. Hugosson, Carlsson, Aus et al., "Mortality Results from the Goteborg Randomised Population-based Prostate-Cancer Screening Trial."

29. "Screening for Prostate Cancer," *UpToDate*, March 2, 2020, https://www.uptodate.com/contents/screening-for-prostate-cancer.

30. Schröder, Hugosson, Carlsson et al., "Screening for Prostate Cancer Decreases the Risk of Developing Metastatic Disease."

31. "Prostate Cancer Screening," United States Preventive Services Task Force, May 8, 2018, https://www.uspreventiveservicestaskforce.org/Page/Document/RecommendationStatementFinal/prostate-cancer-screening.

32. Ibid.

33. "Prostate Cancer Screening," American Family Physician, October 15, 2015, https://www.aafp.org/afp/2015/1015/p683.html.

34. "Annual Screening for Prostate Cancer Did Not Reduce Mortality from Prostate Cancer," *American College of Physicians*, June 16, 2009, http://annals.org/aim/article-abstract/744408/annual-screening-prostate-cancer-did-reduce-mortality-from-prostate-cancer.

35. H. Ballentine Carer, C. Albertsen, J. Barry Michael et. al., "Early Detection of Prostate Cancer: AUA Guidelines," American Urological Association, p. 1.

36. "Should I Get Screened for Prostate Cancer," Centers for Disease Control, July 31, 2019, https://www.cdc.gov/cancer/prostate/basic_info/get -screened.htm.

37. "The Canadian Task Force on Preventive Health Care Recommends Against Screening for Prostate Cancer with the PSA Test," accessed July 12, 2020, https://canadiantaskforce.ca/tools-resources/prostate-cancer-harms -and-benefits/.

38. "Screening," Cancer Research UK, May 31, 2020, http://www.cancer researchuk.org/about-cancer/prostate-cancer/getting-diagnosed/screening.

39. "PSA Testing," UK National Health Service, June 12, 2021, https:// www.nhs.uk/conditions/prostate-cancer/psa-testing/.

40. "Prostate Cancer Screening," Aetna Clinical Policy Bulletin, no. 0521, accessed July 13, 2020, http://www.aetna.com/cpb/medical/data/500_599/0521 .html.

41. "Prostate Cancer Treatment," CIGNA Health Insurance, https://www .cigna.com/individuals-families/health-wellness/hw/medical-topics/prostate -cancer-treatment-ncicdr0000062910.

42. Anthony V. D'Amico, MD, "Prostate Cancer Screening: Who Recommends PSA Testing," Brigham Health Hub, accessed July 13, 2020, https:// brighamhealthhub.org/prevention/prostate-cancer-screening-who-recommends -psa-testing.

43. Schröder, Hugosson, Carlsson et al., "Screening for Prostate Cancer Decreases the Risk of Developing Metastatic Disease."

44. "Prostate Cancer Screening," Aetna Clinical Policy Bulletin, no. 0521.

Chapter 10

1. Eric Klein, ed., Management of Prostate Cancer (Current Clinical Urology) (Totowa, NJ: Humana Press, 2004), 481–89.

2. NCI-Designated Cancer Centers, National Cancer Institute, updated June 24, 2019, https://www.cancer.gov/research/nci-role/cancer-centers.

3. Sidney Kimmel Comprehensive Cancer Center, Prostate Cancer Multidisciplinary Clinic, Johns Hopkins University, August 2019, https://www .hopkinsmedicine.org/kimmel_cancer_center/.

4. Humantis Research Hospital, accessed July 13, 2020, https://www .humanitas.net/?s=considered+one+of+the+most+technologically+advanced+ hospitals+in+Europe&post_type=any.

5. "Why Humanitas," Humanitis Research Hospital, May 2019, https:// www.humanitas.net/why-humanitas/.

6. Nancy E. Epstein, "Multidisciplinary In-hospital Teams Improve Patient Outcomes: A Review," US National Library of Medicine, National

Institutes of Health, August 28, 2014, https://www.ncbi.nlm.nih.gov/pmc/articles/PMC4173201/.

7. Dr. Sean Cavanaugh, Cancer Treatment Centers of America, Chief of Radiation Oncology, https://www.cancercenter.com/physician-directory/sean-cavanaugh.

8. "Prostate Cancer Treatments," University of California San Francisco Health, accessed July 13, 2020, https://www.ucsfhealth.org/conditions/prostate_cancer/treatment.html.

9. "Patient's Guide to Prostate Cancer: Treatments," University of California San Francisco Health, accessed November 20, 2020, https://www.ucsfhealth.org/education/patients_guide_to_prostate_cancer/treatments/.

10. "Laparoscopic Prostatectomy," Cleveland Clinic Health Library, accessed November 20, 2020, https://my.clevelandclinic.org/health/treatments/17160-laparoscopic-prostatectomy.

11. "Prostate Cancer: Laparoscopic Prostate Survey," *Web*MD, December 2019, https://www.webmd.com/prostate-cancer/guide/laparoscopic-prostate-surgery#1.

12. Ibid.

13. "Intensity-modulated Radiation Therapy (IMRT)," Mayo Clinic, accessed September 10, 2020, https://www.mayoclinic.org/tests-procedures/intensity-modulated-radiation-therapy/about/pac-20385147.

14. "Patient's Guide to Prostate Cancer: Treatments," University of California San Francisco Health.

15. Ibid.

16. "Prostate Cancer Cryosurgery Treatment," Columbia University Department of Urology, Irving Medical Center, accessed July 13, 2020, http://columbiaurology.org/adult-urology/urologic-oncology/prostate-cancer/prostate-cancer-cryosurgery-treatment.

17. "Prostate Cancer & Its Treatment," Section VI Treatment Options, University of California San Francisco, accessed September 10, 2020, https://campuslifeservices.ucsf.edu/dmx/PatientEd/SDURO0080.pdf.

18. "Androgen," Encyclopedia Britannica, accessed November 20, 2020, https://www.britannica.com/science/androgen.

19. "Hormone Therapy for Prostate Cancer," American Cancer Society, April 21, 2019, https://www.cancer.org/cancer/prostate-cancer/treating/hormone-therapy.html.

20. "Patient's Guide to Prostate Cancer: Treatments," University of California San Francisco Health.

21. Ibid.

22. Matthew R. Smith, Fred Saad, Simon Chudhury, Stephane Oudard et al., "Apalutamide Treatment and Metastasis-free Survival in Prostate Cancer,"

New England Journal of Medicine, April 12, 2018, http://www.nejm.org/doi/full/10.1056/NEJMoa1715546.

23. Jim Daley, "Prostate Cancer: Surgical Castration Linked to Fewer Adverse Events Than Chemical Castration" Cancer Therapy Advisor, January 21, 2016, https://www.cancertherapyadvisor.com/prostate-cancer/prostate-cancer-surgery-castration-fewer-adverse-events-chemical-treatment/article/466610/.

24. "Patient's Guide to Prostate Cancer: Treatments," University of California San Francisco Health.

25. Nick Mulcahy, "Prostate Cancer Treatments," May 6, 2019, University of California San Francisco Health, https://www.ucsfhealth.org/conditions/prostate_cancer/treatment.html.

26. "In NYC Subway, CyberKnife Prostate Cancer Ads Mislead," MedScape, May 7, 2019, https://www.medscape.com/viewarticle/912619.

27. "Prostate Cancer Treatment by Stage," Beth Israel Deaconess Medical Center, accessed July 13, 2020, https://www.bidmc.org/centers-and-departments/cancer-center/cancer-center-programs-and-services/prostate-cancer-center/prostate-cancer-treatment-options.

Chapter 11

1. "Metacure Trial: Can We Cure More Oligometastatic Prostate Cancer?" Consult QD, Cleveland Clinic, January 13, 2020, https://consultqd.clevelandclinic.org/metacure-trial-can-we-cure-more-oligometastatic-prostate-cancer/.

2. "What Are Late Stage Prostate Cancer Symptoms, What Are Late-Stage Prostate Cancer Symptoms," Prostate.net, January 17, 2019, https://prostate.net/what-are-late-stage-prostate-cancer-symptoms/

3. Ibid.

4. Ibid.

5. Matthew R. Smith, Fred Saad, Simon Chowdhury, Stephane Oudard et al., "Apalutamide Treatment and Metastasis-Free Survival in Prostate Cancer," *New England Journal of Medicine*, April 12, 2018, http://www.nejm.org/doi/full/10.1056/NEJMoa1715546.

6. Marla Paul, "Metastatic Prostate Cancer Cases Way Up: Increase May Be Due to More Lax Screening or More Aggressive Disease," Northwestern Now, July 19, 2016, https://news.northwestern.edu/stories/2016/07/metastatic-prostate-cancer-cases-skyrocket.

7. A. B. Weiner, R. S. Matulewicz, S. E. Eggener, and E. M. Schaeffer, "Increasing Incidence of Prostate Cancer in the United States (2004–2013)," Department of Urology, Northwestern University Feinberg School of Medicine, Chicago, Illinois, July 19, 2016, https://www.nature.com/articles/pcan201630.

8. Jim C. Hu, Paul, Nguyen, Jialin Mao et al., "Increase in Prostate Cancer Distant Metastases at Diagnosis in the United States," Research Letter, Journal of the American Medical Association, May 2017, https://jamanetwork.com/journals/jamaoncology/article-abstract/2594540.

9. Jim Hu, "Incidence of Metastatic Prostate Cancer in Older Men Increases Following Drop in PSA Screening," Weill Cornell School of Medicine, "Newsroom," December 29, 2016, https://news.weill.cornell.edu/news/2016/12/incidence-of-metastatic-prostate-cancer-in-older-men-increases-following-drop-in-psa.

Chapter 12

1. "Cancer and Sex: Why is Nobody Talking About It?" *Newsweek*, July 17, 2017, http://www.newsweek.com/2017/07/28/cancer-sex-life-saving-treatments-havoc-intimacy-638396.html.

Chapter 13

1. Danil V. Makarov, Kristin Chrouser, John L. Gore, Jodi Maranchie et al., "AUA White Paper on Implementation of Shared Decision Making into Urological Practice," ScienceDirect, September 5, 2006, http://www.sciencedirect.com/science/article/pii/S2352077915002733.

2. Paul K. J. Han, Sarah Kobrin, Nancy Breen, Dienaba A. Joseph et al., "National Evidence on the Use of Shared Decision Making in Prostate-Specific Antigen Screening," Annals of Family Medicine, July 2013, https://www.ncbi.nlm.nih.gov/pmc/articles/PMC3704490/ .

3. H. B. Carter, P. C. Albertsen, M. J. Barry et al., "Early Detection of Prostate Cancer (2018)," *American Urological Association*, http://www.auanet.org/guidelines/prostate-cancer-early-detection-guideline.

4. Ibid.

5. "Toward the 'Tipping Point': Decision Aids and Informed," *Health Affairs*, May/June 2007, https://www.healthaffairs.org/author/O%27Connor%2C+Annette+M.

6. "International Patient Decision Aid Standards Collaboration," updated May 31, 2019, http://ipdas.ohri.ca.

7. "About us," Cochran.org, accessed July 13, 2020, http://www.cochrane.org/about-us.

8. "Early Detection of Prostate Cancer," American Urological Association Policy Implications, November 20, 2020, http://www.auanet.org/guidelines/early-detection-of-prostate-cancer-(2013-reviewed-and-validity-confirmed-2015).

9. Ibid.

10. "Advanced Prostate Cancer and Your Relationship," *Web*MD, accessed November 20, 2020, https://www.webmd.com/prostate-cancer/advanced-prostate-cancer-16/prostate-cancer-palliative-care.

11. "Sexual Health, Intimacy and Cancer," Dana-Farber Cancer Institute, Counseling, Health Library, accessed July 13, 2020, https://www.dana-farber.org.

12. "Prostate Cancer, Diagnosis, Coping and Support," Mayo Clinic, May 2019, https://www.mayoclinic.org/diseases-conditions/prostate-cancer/diagnosis-treatment/drc-20353093.

13. "Psycho-Oncology," University of California San Francisco Health, accessed November 20, 2020.

Chapter 14

1. D. Wittman, L. Northouse, S. Foley, D. P. Wood, Jr. et al., "The Psychosocial Aspects of Sexual Recovery After Prostate Cancer Treatment," *International Journal of Impotence Research*, January 22, 2009, https://www.nature.com/articles/ijir200866.

2. "Message on Prostate Surgery Results Not Getting Through," MedPage Today, August 10, 2011, "https://www.medpagetoday.com/hematologyoncology/prostatecancer/27977.

3. Ibid.

4. "Pre-op Counseling for Prostate Surgery Not Effective," Web Physicians blog, January 2012, http://urology.webphysicians.org/2012/01/03/pre-op-counseling-for-prostate-surgery-not-effective/.

5. "Advanced Prostate Cancer and Your Relationship," *Web*MD, July 13, 2020, https://www.webmd.com/prostate-cancer/advanced-prostate-cancer-16/relationship-intimacy.

6. "Preserving Intimacy After Prostate Cancer," Hutch New Stories, May 13, 2014, Fred Hutch Cancer Research Center, https://www.fredhutch.org/en/news/center-news/2014/05/Intimacy-after-prostate-cancer.html.

7. Mehrdad Alemozaffar, Meredith M. Regan, Matthew R. Cooperberg et al., "Prediction of Erectile Function Following Treatment for Prostate Cancer," *Journal of the American Medical Association*, September 21, 2011, https://jamanetwork.com/journals/jama/fullarticle/1104401.

8. Rick Redner, "8 Reasons Why Sexual Desire Is Reduced After Prostate Surgery," Prostate Cancer News Today, August 4, 2017, https://prostatecancernewstoday.com/2017/08/04/prostate-cancer-surgery-eight-reasons-why-sexual-desire-is-reduced/.

Chapter 15

1. Abigail Jones, "Sex and Cancer: Why Is Nobody Talking About It?" *Newsweek*, July 17, 2017, http://www.newsweek.com/2017/07/28/cancer-sex-l ife-saving-treatments-havoc-intimacy-638396.html.

2. Roxanne Nelson, "Preserving Intimacy After Prostate Cancer," "Hutch News Stories," May 13, 2014, https://www.fredhutch.org/en/news/center -news/2014/05/Intimacy-after-prostate-cancer.html.

3. Don. S. Dizon, "What About Intimacy?" ASCO Connection, December 5, 2014, https://connection.asco.org/blogs/what-about-intimacy.html.

4. "Prostate Cancer and Relationships: The Partner's Story, Harvard Perspective on Prostate Cancer," August 2009, http://www.health.harvard.edu/ newsletter_article/Prostate-cancer-and-relationships-The-partners-story.

5. Dizon, "What About Intimacy?"

6. Ashwini C. Bapat, "At Life's End, the Gift of Intimacy," Cognoscenti, WBUR-FM, May 14, 2019, https://www.wbur.org/cognoscenti/2019/05.04/ pallative-care-dying-ashwini-bapat.

Chapter 16

1. Melissa T. Sanford, Kirsten L. Greene, and Peter R. Carroll, "The Argument for Palliative Care in Prostate Cancer," *Translational Andrology and Urology* 2, no. 4 (December 2013), https://tau.amegroups.com/article/ view/2970.

2. Pippa Hawley, "Barriers to Access to Palliative Care," Palliative Care: Research and Treatment, February 20, 2017, https://www.ncbi.nlm.nih.gov/ pmc/articles/PMC5398324.

3. "Palliative Care," World Health Organization, accessed July 13, 2020, http://www.who.int/cancer/palliative/definition/en/.

4. "Palliative Care for Advanced Prostate Cancer," *Web*MD, accessed July 13, 2020, https://www.webmd.com/prostate-cancer/prostate-cancer -pallative-care#1.

5. Ibid.; Sanford, Greene, and Carroll, "The Argument for Palliative Care in Prostate Cancer."

Chapter 17

1. Abigail Jones, "Cancer and Sex: Why Is Nobody Talking About It?" *Newsweek*, July 17, 2017, http://www.newsweek.com/2017/07/28/cancer-sex-l ife-saving-treatments-havoc-intimacy-638396.html.

2. "Leaving My Husband 4 Years After Prostate Cancer," MedHelp, November 22, 2009, https://www.medhelp.org/posts/Relationships/leaving-my -husband-4yrs-after-prostate-cancer/show/1108395.

3. Jones, "Cancer and Sex: Why Is Nobody Talking About It?"

4. "Dealing with Erectile Dysfunction," University of California Los Angeles Health, "Educational Materials," accessed July 18, 2020, https://www.ucla health.org/urology/prostate-cancer/dealing-with-erectile-dysfunction#How MayErectileDysfunctionAffectMySexualRelationships.

5. "Prostate Cancer Counseling Helps Couples' Sex Lives, Says Study," ABC News, September 26, 2011, http://abcnews.go.com/Health/prostate -cancer-study-finds-couples-counseling-helps-restore/story?id=14592459.

6. Jennifer Goodwin, "Couples Counseling Boosts Sex Lives After Prostate Cancer," HealthDay, September 26, 2011, https://consumer.healthday.com/ cancer-information-5/mis-cancer-news-102/couples-counseling-boosts-sex -lives-after-prostate-cancer-657217.html.

7. Dr. Bruce R. Gilbert, Northwell Health, May 2019, https://www.north well.edu/find-care/find-a-doctor/urology/dr-bruce-r-gilbert-md-11308199.

Chapter 18

1. Recurrence, ZERO Cancer.org, accessed July 13, 2020, https://zerocan cer.org/learn/survivors/recurrence/.

2. Michael Kolodziej, "Management of Biochemically Recurrent Prostate Cancer Following Local Therapy," *American Journal of Managed Care*, January 8, 2015, https://www.ajmc.com/journals/supplement/2014/ ace021_dec14_prostate_ce/ace021_dec14_prostatece_kolodziej.

3. "Recurrent Prostate Cancer," *Texas Oncology*, accessed July 13, 2020, https://www.texasoncology.com/types-of-cancer/prostate-cancer/recurrent -prostate-cancer.

4. "Treating Prostate Cancer That Doesn't Go Away or Comes Back After Treatment," American Cancer Society, accessed July 13, 2020, https://www .cancer.org/cancer/prostate-cancer/treating/recurrence.html.

5. "Recurrent Prostate Cancer," *Texas Oncology*.

6. Christopher Sweeney, Yu-Hul Chen, Michael Anthony Carducci, Glenn Liu et al., "Impact on Overall Survival with Chemohormonal Therapy Versus Hormonal Therapy for Hormone-Sensitive Newly Metastatic Prostate Cancer: An ECOG-led Phase III Randomized Trial," *Journal of Clinical Oncology* 32, no. 18, https://ascopubs.org/doi/abs/10.1200/jco.2014.32.18_suppl.lba2.

7. I. Tannock, R. de Wit, W. Berry et al., "Docetaxel plus Prednisone or Mitoxantrone plus Prednisone for Advanced Prostate Cancer," *New England*

Journal of Medicine, October 7, 2004: 1502–512, https://pubmed.ncbi.nlm.nih .gov/15470213/.

8. E. Basch, K. Autio, C. J. Ryan et al., "Abiraterone Acetate plus Prednisone Versus Prednisone Alone in Chemotherapy-naive Men with Metastatic Castration-resistant Prostate Cancer: Patient-Reported Outcome Results of a Randomized Phase 3 Trial," *The Lancet Oncology*, September 25, 2013, https:// www.thelancet.com/journals/lanonc/article/PIIS1470-2045(13)70424-8/ fulltext.

9. "Recurrent Prostate Cancer," *Texas Oncology*.

10. P. W. Kantoff, C. S. Higano, N. D. Shore et al., "Sipuleucel-T Immunotherapy for Castration-Resistant Prostate Cancer," *New England Journal of Medicine*, July 29, 2010.

11. "Pharmaco-economic Aspects of Sipuleucel-T Abstract," 2010 Genitourinary Cancers Symposium, *Urology Today*, April 6, 2012, https:// www.urotoday.com/recent-abstracts/urologic-oncology/prostate-cancer/49705 -pharmaco-economic-aspects-of-sipuleucel-t-abstract.html.

12. Sonya J. Snedecor, John A. Carter, Satyin Kaura, and Marc F. Botteman, "Denosumab versus Zoledronic Acid for Treatment of Bone Metastases in Men with Castration-Resistant Prostate Cancer: A Cost-Effectiveness Analysis," *Journal of Medical Economics*, Taylor Francis Online, June 29, 2012, https:// www.tandfonline.com/doi/full/10.3111/13696998.2012.719054.

13. "Immunotherapy: A Vaccine for Prostate Cancer," Prostate Cancer Foundation," June 15, 2017, https://www.pcf.org/news/immunotherapy-a -vaccine-for-prostate-cancer/.

14. Matthew R. Smith, Fred Saad, Robert Coleman et al., "Denosumab and Bone-Metastasis-Free Survival in Men with Castration-Resistant Prostate Cancer: Results of a Phase 3, Randomized, Placebo-Controlled Trial," *The Lancet*, November 16, 2011, https://www.thelancet.com/journals/lancet/article/ PIIS0140-6736(11)61226-9/fulltext.

Chapter 19

1. "Psychosocial Case Is a Critical Component of Value-based Oncology," *The ASCO Post*, May 10 2019, https://www.ascopost.com/issues/may-10-2019/ psychosocial-care-is-a-critical-component-of-value-based-oncology.

2. USTOO.com, https://www.ustoo.org.

Chapter 20

1. "Cancer Fatigues," Cleveland Clinic, accessed November 17, 2020, https://my.clevelandclinic.org/health/diseases/5230-cancer-fatigue http://chemocare.com/chemotherapy/side-effects/fatigue-and-cancer.aspx.

2. Ibid.

3. "How Can I Manage Fatigue," ZERO Cancer.org, May 2019, https://zerocancer.org/learn/current-patients/side-effects/fatigue/.

4. Andrew Chesler, "The Importance of Identifying Anxiety and Depression in Men with Prostate Cancer," *Oncology Nursing News*, September 13, 2018, https://www.oncnursingnews.com/contributor/cancer-care/2018/09/the-importance-of-identifying-anxiety-and-depression-in-men-with-prostate-cancer.

5. Ibid.

6. "What Will I Learn by Reading This?" Educational Materials, University of California Los Angeles Health, accessed July 18, 2020, https://www.uclahealth.org/urology/prostate-cancer/dealing-with-erectile-dysfunction.

7. "Dealing with Erectile Dysfunction," University of California Los Angeles Health, July 2019, http://urology.ucla.edu/prostate-cancer/dealing-with-erectile-dysfunction.

8. Dr. Ananya Mandal, "Semen Physiology," News-Medical Life Science, Updated February 27, 2019, https://www.news-medical.net/health/Semen-Physiology.aspx.

9. "Types of Urinary Incontinence," Harvard Health Publishing, December 2014, https://www.health.harvard.edu/bladder-and-bowel/types-of-urinary-incontinence.

10. "A patient's story: Overcoming incontinence," March 11, 2009, Harvard Health Blog, https://www.health.harvard.edu/blog/a-patients-story-overcoming-incontinence-2009031125.

11. "What Is the Prostate's Role in Urination?" Cleveland Clinic, accessed July 13, 2020, https://my.clevelandclinic.org/health/treatments/8096-prostate-cancer-urinary-incontinence-after-surgery.

12. Dana Jennings, "Living with Incontinence After Prostate Cancer," *New York Times*, March 3, 2009, https://well.blogs.nytimes.com/2009/03/03/living-with-incontinence-after-prostate-cancer/.

13. "Urinary Incontinence in Men," MedicineNet, May 2019, https://www.medicinenet.com/urinary_incontinence/article.htm#urinary_incontinence_ui_in_men_facts.

14. "What Are Kegels, and Why Should I Do Them," *Web*MD, accessed July 13, 2020, https://www.webmd.com/women/guide/kegels-should-i-do-them.

15. "How Is Urinary Incontinence in Men Treated?" MedicineNet, May 2019, https://www.medicinenet.com/urinary_incontinence/article.htm#how_is_urinary_incontinence_ui_in_men_treated.

16. "Prostate Cancer: Urinary Incontinence After Surgery: Procedure Details," Cleveland Clinic, June 2019, https://my.clevelandclinic.org/health/treatments/8096-prostate-cancer-urinary-incontinence-after-surgery/procedure-details.

17. "Bowel Incontinence (Fecal Incontinence)" MedicineNet, May 2019, https://www.medicinenet.com/fecal_incontinence/article.htm.

18. "Bowel Dysfunction After Prostate Cancer Treatment," "Health," Johns Hopkins University, accessed January 15, 2021, https://www.hopkinsmedicine.org/health/treatment-tests-and-therapies/bowel-dysfunction-after-prostate-cancer-treatment.

19. Yasuko Maeda, "Fecal Incontinence Following Radiotherapy for Prostate Cancer: A Systematic Review," National Center for Biotechnology Information, PubMed.gov, February 2011, https://www.ncbi.nlm.nih.gov/pubmed/21257215.

20. Joseph Brownstein, "Prostate Cancer Diagnosis May Bring Suicide, Heart Risks," ABC News, December 15, 2009, https://abcnews.go.com/Health/ProstateCancerNews/prostate-cancer-diagnosis-brings-suicide-heart-risk/story?id=9333628.

Chapter 21

1. "Erectile Dysfunction After Prostate Cancer," "Health," Johns Hopkins Medicine, August 2019, accessed July 15, 2020, https://www.hopkinsmedicine.org/health/conditions-and-diseases/prostate-cancer/erectile-dysfunction-after-prostate-cancer.

2. "New Options for Treating Erectile Dysfunction," Harvard Health Publishing, March 11, 2009, https://www.harvardprostateknowledge.org/new-options-for-treating-erectile-dysfunction.

3. "Erectile Dysfunction After Prostate Surgery," "Health," Johns Hopkins Medicine.

4. "9 Popular Ways to Treat Erectile Dysfunction," Everyday Health, August 2019, https://www.everydayhealth.com/erectile-dysfunction-pictures/popular-ways-to-treat-erectile-dysfunction.aspx.

5. Dr. J. Francios Eid, "Penile Injection Therapy Highlights," Advanced Urological Care P.C., https://www.urologicalcare.com/erectile-dysfunction/penile-injection-therapy/.

6. Ibid.

7. "Comparing Implant Types," Penile Implants, Mayo Clinic, accessed November 17, 2020, https://www.mayoclinic.org/tests-procedures/penile-implants/about/pac-20384916.

8. Dr. Andrew J. Roth et al., "Prostate Cancer: Quality of Life, Psychosocial Implications and Treatment Choices," August 4, 2008, US National Library of PMC/NCBI, https://www.ncbi.nlm.nih.gov/pmc/articles/PMC2796196/.

Chapter 22

1. "What Is the Prostate Gland, Conditions Affecting the Prostate," Medical News Today, January 11, 2018, https://www.medicalnewstoday.com/articles/319859.php.

2. Dr. Amaya Mandal, "Semen Psychology," Medical Life Sciences, July 2019, https://www.news-medical.net/health/Semen-Physiology.aspx.

3. "What Are Early Symptoms of Prostate Cancer," Healthline.com, March 28, 2017, https://www.healthline.com/health/prostate-cancer-symptoms#urinary-symptoms.

4. "How Does the Prostate Work?" InformedHealth.org, National Institutes of Health, August 23, 2016, https://www.ncbi.nlm.nih.gov/books/NBK279291/.

Chapter 23

1. George Orwell, Animal Farm, GoodReads.com, accessed November 17, 2020, https://www.goodreads.com/quotes/6466-all-animals-are-equal-but-some-animals-are-more-equal.

2. Harvard University, 2017 Annual Report on Prostate Cancer, 2018, 35.

3. Molika Ashford, "What Does the Prostate Gland Do? "Life's Little Mysteries," August 9, 2010, https://www.livescience.com/32751-what-does-the-prostate-gland-do.html.

4. "Inherited Risk for Prostate Cancer," https://www.mskcc.org/cancer-care/risk-assessment-screening/hereditary-genetics/genetic-counseling/inherited-risk-prostate.

5. "BRCA2 Gene," National Institutes of Health, July 7, 2020, https://ghr.nlm.nih.gov/gene/BRCA2.

6. John von Radowitz, "Tall Men Are More Likely to Develop Prostate Cancer, New Research Suggests," The Independent, July 13, 2017, https://www.independent.co.uk/life-style/health-and-families/health-news/prostate-cancer-tall-men-increased-risk-disease-death-tumours-height-correlation-oxford-university-a7838481.html.

7. "Prostate Cancer: Additional Facts for African American Men and Their Families," Prostate Cancer Foundation, accessed July 15, 2020, https://

res.cloudinary.com/pcf/image/upload/v1553031384/AfAm_PCaInfoGuide
-031919_dygfjz.pdf.

8. Nick Mulcahy, "Blacks, Whites Similar Survival in Advanced Prostate Cancer, But. . ." Medscape, Oncology News, February 27, 2019, https://www.medscape.com/viewarticle/909643.

9. Lisa Rapaport, "Blacks with Prostate Cancer Less Likely to Get Ideal Treatment," Reuters, August 2, 2017, https://www.reuters.com/article/us-pros tate-treatment-race/blacks-with-prostate-cancer-less-likely-to-get-ideal-treat ment-idUSKCN1B32E6.

10. Hugh McIntosh, "Why Do African American Men Suffer More Prostate Cancer?" *Journal of the National Cancer Institute*, February 5, 1997, https://academic.oup.com/jnci/article/89/3/188/2526672.

11. "Prostate Cancer Risk Factors," American Cancer Society, https://www.cancer.org/cancer/prostate-cancer/early-detection/risk-factors-for-prostate-cancer.html.

12. M. Quinn and P. Babb, "Patterns and Trends in Prostate Cancer Incidence, Survial, Prevalence, and Mortality, Part 1: International Comparisons," BJUI International, June 24, 2002, https://bjui-journals.onlinelibrary.wiley.com/doi/abs/10.1046/j.1464-410X.2002.2822.x.

13. "Our Analysis of Worldwide Research on Prostate Cancer," World Cancer Research Fund International, accessed March 16, 2021, https://res.cloudinary.com/pcf/image/upload/v1575394191/WellnessGuide_interactive_rev12.2.19_yrdiph.pdf.

14. Danish Mazhar, "Diet and Prostate Cancer," accessed July 15, 2020, https://www.usnews.com/news/best-countries/articles/2019-02-04/australia-has-the-highest-rates-of-cancer-worldwide-analysis-shows.

15. Miranda R. Jones, Corinne E. Joshu, Norma Kanarek, Ana Navas-Acien et al., "Cigarette Smoking and Prostate Cancer Mortality in Four US States, 1999–2010," Centers for Disease Control, April 14, 2016, https://www.cdc.gov/pcd/issues/2016/15_0454.htm.

Chapter 24

1. "Prostate Cancer Prevention: Ways to Reduce Your Risk," Mayo Clinic, November 6, 2018, https://www.mayoclinic.org/diseases-conditions/prostate-cancer/in-depth/prostate-cancer-prevention/art-20045641.

2. "The Science of Living Well," Prostate Cancer Foundation, November 6, 2019, https://res.cloudinary.com/pcf/image/upload/v1574120581/Well nessGuide_interactive_rev11.15.19_goostr.pdf.

3. "Centers for Disease Control and Prevention HPV and Men—Fact Sheet," December 28, 2016, https://www.cdc.gov/std/hpv/stdfact-hpv-and-men.htm.

4. "Can Prostate Cancer Be Prevented?" American Cancer Society, accessed July 15, 2020, https://www.cancer.org/cancer/prostate-cancer/early-detection/prevention.html.

5. "The Science of Living Well, Beyond Cancer," Prostate Cancer Foundation, 2019, https://res.cloudinary.com/pcf/image/upload/v1574120581/WellnessGuide_interactive_rev11.15.19_goostr.pdf.

6. Ibid, 89.

7. "Flip the Switch," Harvard Medical School, January 15, 2018, accessed November 17, 2020, https://hms.harvard.edu/news/flip-switch#.WmAO302sF34.mailto.

8. Bill Nelson, "Prostate Cancer and Diet," Prostate Cancer Update, vol. 5 (Winter 2000), James Buchanan Brady Urological Institute, Johns Hopkins University, http://urology.jhu.edu/newsletter/prostate_cancer512.php.

9. "Your Diet and Physical Activity," Prostate Cancer UK, accessed July 15, 2020, https://prostatecanceruk.org/prostate-information/living-with-prostate-cancer/your-diet-and-physical-activity.

10. "A Case-Control Study of Diet and Prostate Cancer in Japan; Possible Protective Effect of Traditional Japanese Diet," *Cancer Science*, Wiley Online Library, August 19, 2005, https://onlinelibrary.wiley.com/doi/abs/10.1111/j.1349-7006.2004.tb02209.x.

11. "Charred Foods Bad, Veggies Good," Discovery, Johns Hopkins Medicine," January 22, 2016, https://www.hopkinsmedicine.org/brady-urology-institute/patient-information/books-publications/articles/charred-food-bad-veggies-good-for-the-prostate.

12. "Sulforaphane: Benefits, Side Effects, and Food Sources," Healthline, February 26, 2019, https://www.healthline.com/nutrition/sulforaphane.

13. "The Science of Living Well, Beyond Cancer," Prostate Cancer Foundation.

14. "Starving Prostate Cancer with What You Eat: Apple Peels, Red Grapes, Turmeric," *Science Daily*, June 6, 2017, https://www.sciencedaily.com/releases/2017/06/170606112750.htm.

15. "Eating Mushrooms May Help Lower Prostate Cancer," *Science Daily*, September 5, 2009, https://www.sciencedaily.com/releases/2019/09/190905080106.htm.

16. "So, What Are Some Different Types of Mushrooms?" Mushroom Appreciation.com, accessed July 15, 2020, https://www.mushroom-appreciation.com/types-of-mushrooms.html#sthash.UQal4Vud.yJqV63I8.dpbs.

17. "Healthy Grilling: Reducing the Risk of Cancer," Cedars Sinai blog, July 30, 2018, https://www.cedars-sinai.org/blog/grilling-cancer-risk.html.

18. Sheldon Marks, "Is There a Prostate Cancer Diet?" *Web*MD, accessed November 11, 2020, https://www.webmd.com/prostate-cancer/features/is-there -prostate-cancer-diet.

19. "Pomegranate Juice: A Cure for Prostate Cancer?" Mayo Clinic, accessed July 15, 2020, https://www.mayoclinic.org/diseases-conditions/ prostate-cancer/expert-answers/pomegranate-juice/faq-20058204.

20. "Diet and Weight Loss: Which Has More Sugar," reviewed by Kathleen Zelman, October 22, 2018, https://www.medicinenet.com/diet_weight_loss _sugar/article.htm?ecd=mnl_spc_071819.

Chapter 25

1. "What Is Metastatic Prostate Cancer?" *Web*MD, accessed July 15, 2020, https://www.webmd.com/prostate-cancer/advanced-prostate-cancer-16/ metastatic-prostate-cancer.

2. "Metastatic Cancer: When Cancer Spreads," National Cancer Institute, accessed July 15, 2020, https://www.cancer.gov/types/metastatic-cancer.

3. "What Happens When Prostate Cancer Spread to the Bones?" Healthline, accessed July 15, 2020, https://www.healthline.com/health/prostate-cancer -prognosis-life-expectancy-bone-metastases.

Index

abdominal surgery, 201
Abiraterone Zytiga®, 113, 167
ablation, 61
active surveillance, 29, 33–34, 38,
    45, 49, 50, 103–104, 115, 166
adenocarcinoma, 23
adjuvant hormone therapy, 53
adrenal glands, 98, 113, 167, 234
ADT. *See* Androgen Deprivation
    Therapy
advanced prostate cancer. *See*
    prostate cancer
Advanced Urologic Care, P.C., 198
Aetna Insurance, 81, 83
Affordable Care Act, 30, 35
African American men, 11, 13, 17,
    19, 45, 57, 66, 80, 212–14
age, 9, 11, 17, 19, 24, 25, 34–35, 37,
    39–41, 50, 80–82, 92, 137, 184,
    191, 195, 200–201, 205–206,
    209, 211
Alexandria, Virginia, 30
alpha-blockers, 198
Alprostadil, 199–200
alternative therapies, 93, 105, 112
American Academy of Family
    Physicians, 79
American Academy of
    Sexologists, 140
American Cancer Society, 23, 25–26,
    44, 58, 61, 69, 72, 80–81, 98,
    121, 148, 157, 165, 178, 211, 218,
    233, 237
American College of Physicians, 80
American Journal of
    Epidemiology, 209
American Journal of Cancer Care, 23
American Journal of Managed Care,
    151, 163
American Medical Association, 64
American men, 1, 11, 17, 21, 39, 88,
    121, 171, 213, 221, 230
American Society of Clinical
    Oncology, 148, 176, 178, 213
American Urological Association
    (AUA), 25, 30–31, 35, 51, 55–56,
    66, 70–71, 73–75, 80–81, 83, 90,
    110, 125–26, 128;
    Journal of Urology, 77
anal muscles, 62, 190–91, 218
androgen, 98–99, 100, 113, 168, 210;
    blockade, 102;
    Androgen Deprivation Therapy
    (ADT), 33–34, 42, 52, 64, 65,

About the Authors

Harley A. Haynes, MD, is Emeritus Professor of Medicine, Harvard Medical School, and a member of the Department of Dermatology at Massachusetts General Brigham and Women's Hospital and the Dana Farber Cancer Institute. Dr. Haynes has received numerous awards for his outstanding leadership, among them the Daniel D. Federman Outstanding Clinical Educator Award in 2000. The Dermatology Foundation recognized him with their Lifetime Career Educator Award in 2004. Extensively published, Dr. Haynes also influenced the training of dermatology residents for fifty years through his bedside teaching and many contributions to national educational committees and his significant number of teaching materials.

Dr. Haynes was diagnosed with prostate cancer in 2013.

Richard M. Miles has written for numerous publications including *The Birmingham Post-Herald*, *Newsweek* magazine, and *The Atlanta Constitution*. Miles has received numerous awards for his writing and journalistic design work, including two Apex Awards for Publications Excellence, Golden and Silver Flame Awards, and a Gold Mercury International Award, among others. Miles lives in Hilton Head Island, South Carolina.

Mr. Miles was diagnosed with prostate cancer in 2002.